Making Sense of Fibromyalgia

Making Sense of Fibromyalgia

DANIEL J. WALLACE, M.D.

Clinical Professor of Medicine
Cedars-Sinai/UCLA School of Medicine
Los Angeles, California

JANICE BROCK WALLACE, M.P.A.

New York   Oxford
OXFORD UNIVERSITY PRESS
1999

Oxford University Press

Oxford   New York

Athens   Auckland   Bangkok   Bogotá   Bombay
Buenos Aires   Cape Town   Chennai   Dar es Salaam
Delhi   Florence   Hong Kong   Istanbul   Karachi
Kuala Lumpur   Madrid   Melbourne   Mexico City
Mumbai   Nairobi   Paris   São Paulo   Singapore
Taipei   Tokyo   Toronto   Warsaw

and associated companies in
Berlin   Ibadan

Library of Congress Cataloging-in-Publication Data
Wallace, Daniel J. (Daniel Jeffrey), 1949–
Making sense of fibromyalgia / by Daniel J.
Wallace and Janice Brock Wallace
p. cm.   Includes index
ISBN 0-19-511611-9
1. Fibromyalgia—Popular works.
I. Wallace, Janice B.
RC927.3.W34   1998   616.7'4—dc21
98-28531

5 7 9 8 6 4

Printed in the United States of America
on acid-free paper

Contents

Foreword

Making Sense of Fibromyalgia is a well-written compendium directed to the millions with severe fatigue, muscular pain, poor sleep patterns, and the other symptoms characteristic of fibromyalgia. While there is continuing debate in the medical and research community about the causes and treatments for this misunderstood syndrome, Dr. Daniel J. Wallace's clinical experience and studied review of the current literature have enabled him to produce a book that discusses many of the current theories and understandings.

Dr. Wallace's specific discussions on the diagnostic elements; procedures that support, differentiate, and exclude fibromyalgia as a primary or secondary condition; and specific therapies and their expected efficacies continue the learning process for the reader and provide hope through better understanding of this often maligned condition.

This is an important book that provides a nice complement to the Arthritis Foundation's own publication *Your Personal Guide to Living with Fibromyalgia*. The Arthritis Foundation, Southern California Chapter, is grateful to Dr. Daniel J. Wallace and Oxford University Press for their support of our program for people with fibromyalgia through donations from the sale of this book, *Making Sense of Fibromyalgia*.

Medical & Scientific Committee
Arthritis Foundation, Southern California Chapter
Los Angeles, California

Preface

To talk of diseases is a sort of Arabian Night's entertainment
Sir William Osler (1849–1919)

Among the childhood pastimes we enjoyed was a peculiar board game known as "Uncle Wiggily" (Fig. 1). Its premise seems quaint when viewed from an adult perspective some 40 years later, but the first player enabling Uncle Wiggily to reach Doc Possum's house so that his rheumatism could be treated was the winner. Along the way, all sorts of nostrums, barriers, diversions, and misinformation deterred Uncle Wiggily from his goal. What, we asked our child's mind, was *rheumatism*? This mysterious, all-encompassing term could apply to fibromyalgia. Fibromyalgia is a syndrome that defies our usual concepts of a disorder and is classified by the Arthritis Foundation as a form of "soft tissue rheumatism."

The purpose of this monograph is to enable you to help yourself; to make it easier to work with your doctor and other allied health professionals; to improve the way you feel; and to promote a better quality of life. To begin, there are several reasons why fibromyalgia is plagued by misunderstanding:

- Although it is now recognized as a legitimate syndrome by the American Medical Association, American College of Rheumatology, Arthritis Foundation, and American College of Physicians, as well as the World Health Organization, some doctors still question its existence. This is largely a consequence of incomplete medical training that was (and often still is) primarily hospital based. Outpatient (office-based) clinical medicine training, which included fibromyalgia, was largely overlooked. Patients are rarely, if ever, hospitalized for fibromyalgia. Also, statistically validated criteria for defining fibromyalgia were not endorsed by organized medicine until 1990. Many physicians are therefore unaware that fibromyalgia has been accorded its own coding number for insurance billing (7290).
- Fibromyalgia patients often have normal blood tests and imaging studies and are thought by some health care professionals to make up many of their symptoms. Certain doctors consider fibromyalgia patients to be hypochondriacs or seekers of medical attention for purposes of litigation or secondary gain. Fortunately, there are now reproducible tests documenting that these

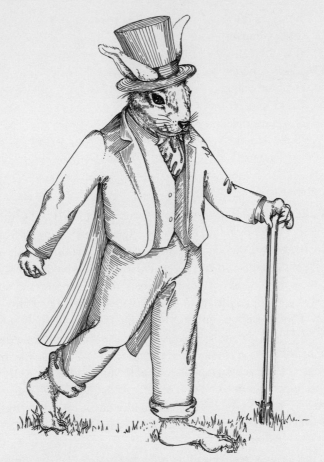

Fig. 1 *An achy Uncle Wiggily on his way to visit Doc Possum.*

complaints are real and studies showing that hypochondriasis is extremely rare in fibromyalgia.

■ Six million Americans meet the criteria for fibromyalgia. On the average, they saw an average of four doctors before they were correctly diagnosed, and many were convinced they had a life-threatening illness such as a body-wide cancer. Fibromyalgia is a combination of pain, fatigue, and systemic symptoms. Ten million patient visits to doctors every year in the United States are for pain; $85 billion is spent annually to diagnose or manage chronic pain, including litigation fees. One group has estimated that patients with fibromyalgia run up $9 billion in medical expenses annually. Additionally, at any visit, 15 percent of all patients tell their doctor they are tired. There is a paucity of reliable, detailed information about the fibromyalgia syndrome that patients can use to help themselves or others.

- Many employers do not realize that fibromyalgia is a treatable workplace problem. It can impair job performance even though its symptoms and signs are invisible. Overall, 700 million work days are lost annually due to pain, and 50 million Americans are partially disabled due to chronic pain. Up to 10 percent of fibromyalgia patients are totally disabled, 30 percent require job modifications, and 30 percent have to change their job in order to remain employed. Appropriate treatment, workstation modifications, and counseling could save the American public hundreds of millions of dollars, improve our productivity, and maintain the self-esteem of the fibromyalgia sufferer.
- Every year, $13 billion is spent out of pocket for non-insurance-reimbursed care by alternative medicine physicians and other caregivers in the United States. Some of this is spent by fibromyalgia patients who are frustrated by the lack of attention, knowledge, and concern of their primary care and specialist physicians.
- In our opinion, there is a relative shortage of rheumatologists, the subspecialists within internal medicine who deal with fibromyalgia, and too little research is ongoing to understand its cause, diagnosis, and treatment. In 1996, the National Institutes of Health allocated only $1 million for fibromyalgia research.

This book is intended not only for fibromyalgia patients, but also for their loved ones, primary care physicians, allied health professionals (nurses, social workers, dentists, physical therapists, psychologists, occupational therapists, vocational rehabilitation counselors, physician assistants, chiropractors, and dietitians), and other people who care about them. We gratefully acknowledge the assistance provided us by Joan Bossert of Oxford University Press, the Arthritis Foundation's Southern California Chapter (especially Lori Port and James Louie, M.D.), Kristin Thorson of the American Fibromyalgia Syndrome Association, Dr. Allan Metzger, Frances Brock, Terri Hoffman for her artwork, Amanda Trujillo, and our children, Naomi, Phillip, and Sarah.

Los Angeles, California   D. J. W.
March 1998   J. B. W.

Fibromyalgia Made Simple: A Parable

Pain has an element of blank;
It cannot recollect
When it began, or if there were
A day when it was not.

It has no future but itself,
Its infinite realms contain
Its past, enlightened to perceive
New periods of pain.
  Emily Dickinson (1830–1896),
  Pain Has an Element of Blank

If you have the chronic pain of fibromyalgia, you may be frustrated by the lack of understanding shown by people around you. This is particularly true of the people you live and work with. If only they could feel for 1 day how you feel all year! Pain has no memory and no mercy. Is it like a bad flu or a severe headache? How can you find the words to describe it? You might wish to recite this short explanation; the next 200 pages provide the details.

Picture your body as being a series of electrical circuits. Suppose that you have the unfortunate tendency to injure your shoulder repeatedly. What happens? As part of a chronic pain response, a wire goes from the shoulder to your spine, and a second wire then travels up the spinal cord to your brain. The brain receives a signal that says, "I hurt my shoulder; let me do something about it." The brain then makes a chemical or chemicals that suppress the pain. It wires a signal back down the spinal column, and a second wire returns to the shoulder. The chemical is released, and the pain gets better or goes away.

What happens in fibromyalgia? Your body becomes "cross-circuited" (Fig. 2). Not only does the body not send the chemical message from the wire to alleviate pain, but instead, pain is amplified. With time, the electrical circuits become "wiry" and excitable. Normally non-painful stimuli are regarded as painful ones. The circuits discharge signals that increase your perception of pain, not only in

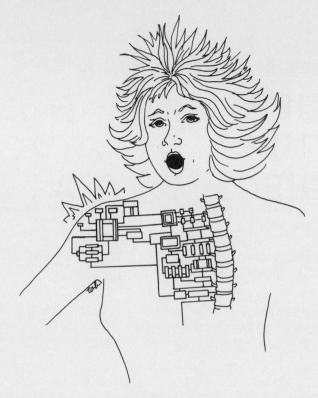

Fig. 2 *Cross-circuiting giving the wrong message after shoulder trauma.*

the region that was hurt but also in the area around it. As a result, the processes that regulate your body become confused and you start to develop all sorts of troublesome symptoms. You can't get a good night's sleep, your muscles go into spasm, and you become fatigued. This aggravates you further and creates a vicious cycle that makes the pain even worse. In a nutshell, this series of events is observed in fibromyalgia.

Let's explore how this happens and what can be done about it.

Part I

THE WHYS AND WHEREFORES OF FIBROMYALGIA

Is it nothing to you, all that pass by? Behold and see. Is there any pain like unto my pain, which is done unto me, wherewith the Lord has afflicted me in the day of his fierce anger? From above, he has sent fire into my bones . . . and I am weary and faint all the day . . .

Jeremiah, in Lamentations 11:12–13

In this part the reader will discover how fibromyalgia evolved and was ultimately defined. Although descriptions of it date back to biblical times, the perception of fibromyalgia as a syndrome represents a convergence of two historical threads: those relating to ongoing musculoskeletal pain (joint and muscle aches) and those dealing with chronic fatigue and a sense of debility. Both official and practical definitions of fibromyalgia will be discussed, and we will consider the number of people who have the syndrome, as well as population groups that most frequently develop it.

1

How Our Understanding of Fibromyalgia Evolved

*. . . and wearisome nights are appointed to me. When I lie
down, I say, When shall I arise, and the night be gone? And I
am full of tossings to and fro unto the dawning of the day . . .
and the days of affliction have taken hold upon me. My
bones are pierced in me in the night season; and my sinews
take no rest.*

Job 7:3–4 and 30:16–17.

There are times when rheumatologists have been accused of making up new syndromes. For example, in the last 15 years, our specialty has described new rheumatic entities including Lyme disease, the musculoskeletal manifestations of acquired immune deficiency syndrome (AIDS), eosinophilic myalgia syndrome (from L-tryptophan contamination), and siliconosis (which, if it exists, results from silicone breast implants). Fibromyalgia is not in this group. Evidence for the syndrome can be found as far back in history as the book of Job, where he complained of "sinews (that) take no rest."

MUSCULOSKELETAL PAIN AMPLIFICATION

Seemingly exaggerated tenderness of the muscles and soft tissues to touch was documented in the 19th-century medical literature by French, German, and British scientists, who called it *spinal irritation*, *Charcot's hysteria*, or a *morbid affection*. The English physician Sir William Gowers coined the term *fibrositis* in 1904 in a paper on lumbago (low back pain) when he tried to describe inflammatory changes in the fibrous tissues of the muscles of the low back. Gowers was wrong. There is no such thing as inflammation of the fibrous tissues, but the term lived on because British physicians used *fibrositis* to denote pain in the upper back and neck areas among Welsh coal miners in the 1920s and 1930s. The definition of fibrositis cross-pollinated during the Second World War when United States, Canadian, Australian, and New Zealand physicians served with their British counterparts. Soldiers who were unwilling to fight or who experienced shell shock, or complained of aches and pains without any obvious disease, were diagnosed as having fibrositis.

A symptom complex of fatigue, palpitations, dizziness, gastrointestinal symptoms, headache, sleep disturbance, and aching was first noted by the Union physician J. M. da Costa among 300 soldiers during the Civil War who had what he termed an "irritable heart." The first mention of fibrositis in the North American medical literature appeared in a rheumatology textbook written by Wallace Graham in 1940. Rheumatology established its first fellowship and training programs in the United States after World War II and, more often than not, their directors were medical officers who had become interested in the discipline as a result of working with their British colleagues.

No substantive changes in the understanding of fibrositis were evident until a series of very important observations were published by the rheumatologist Hugh Smythe and his colleagues at the University of Toronto in the mid-1970s. They renamed the disorder "fibrositis syndrome" and convincingly connected it to systemic symptoms such as fatigue and sleep abnormalities. Smythe popularized the use of the *tender point examination* suggested by others and frequently referred to fibrositis as a *pain amplification disorder*.

FATIGUE SYNDROMES

The history of fibromyalgia is one of merging observations from two directions. Musculoskeletal aches in the soft tissues (supporting areas near muscles and joints) were termed fibrositis and eventually became associated with nonmusculoskeletal symptoms such as fatigue and sleep disorders. From the other direction, fatigue syndromes ultimately were correlated with fibromyalgia. In 1750, Sir Richard Manningham described *febricula* or "little fever," among mostly upper-class females, who were afflicted with "listlessness, with great lassitude and weariness all over the body . . . little flying pains . . . the patient is a little . . . forgetful." These complaints were aggravated by stress.

Dr. George Beard (1839–1883) first used the word *neurasthenia* to describe deficient nerve tone, general debility, poor appetite, and "living on a plane lower than normal." This wonderful Victorian expression characterized many women in English and American literature throughout the 19th century, ranging from Miss Marchmont in Charlotte Brontë's *Villette* to Mrs. Snow in *Polyanna*. Neurasthenia represented a form of "failure to thrive" and often reflected the stunted aspirations of worldly women whose ability to get ahead was blocked by outmoded societal conventions of trying to cope with the Industrial Revolution and the Age of Mechanization. All too frequently, neurasthenia was managed by uptight and condescending male physicians who used a variety of seemingly preposterous remedies such as rest cures, overfeeding, electricity, clitoridectomy, or oophorectomy (removal of the clitoris or ovaries). During World War I, males suffering from shell shock resulting from trench warfare and exhibiting symptoms of neurasthenia were described; thereafter, the term disappeared from the medical literature.

PROLONGED RECOVERY FROM INFECTIOUS ILLNESSES

Between the 1930s and 1950s, patients exposed to infections such as polio during epidemics and a bacterial disease known as *brucellosis* were identified as having postinfectious chronic fatigue, aching, and debility. Other patients were evaluated by neurologists and found to have atypical forms of myasthenia gravis or multiple sclerosis. Some were consequently labeled as having *chronic nervous exhaustion, myasthenic syndrome, Icelandic disease, myalgic encephalomyelitis,* or *epidemic neuromyasthenia,* depending on where and by whom they were treated. The 1980s signaled the advent of *Epstein-Barr virus syndrome,* a postviral fatigue syndrome ultimately renamed *chronic fatigue syndrome.* Chronic fatigue syndrome frequently overlaps with fibromyalgia; this relationship is discussed in Chapter 13.

THE LINKAGE OF PAIN, FATIGUE, DYSREGULATION SPECTRUM SYNDROME, AND POSTINFECTIOUS SYNDROMES

Smythe's connection of fibrositis with systemic symptoms and the inappropriateness of the term *fibrositis* (since no inflammation was present) prompted Dr. Muhammed Yunus and his associates at the University of Illinois at Peoria to take up a suggestion of Dr. Kahler Hench (son of Dr. Phillip Hench, the only rheumatologist to win a Nobel Prize—for discovering that cortisone helped arthritis) that the term *fibromyalgia* better described the syndrome. Yunus was also the first to validate statistically the benefits of measuring tender points and to compare fibromyalgia populations with healthy normal, or control groups. Published in 1981, these observations were immediately endorsed by nearly all rheumatologists. Yunus also was the first investigator to associate objectively what are now called *dysregulation spectrum syndrome* complaints such as irritable colon, tension headache, numbness, tingling, and swelling or edema with the disorder. He also postulated that chemicals creating these symptoms and signs are also influenced by factors such as emotional or physical stress or trauma, mood, and behavior.

During the 1980s, studies showed that patients diagnosed with fibromyalgia included many originally described as having conditions such as muscular rheumatism, musculoligamentous strain, and other syndromes diagnosed by orthopedists, neurologists, neurosurgeons, and physical medicine specialists. Further, the development of tests supporting scientifically acceptable, reproducible abnormalities in fibromyalgia led the American Medical Association in 1987 to editorialize that the syndrome truly existed. A committee subsequently was formed to devise a definition and description of fibromyalgia for statistical and research purposes, and these criteria were adopted by the American College of Rheumatology in 1990.

SUMMING UP

A biblical description of a set of symptoms and signs culminated in the recognition of a syndrome characterized by musculoskeletal complaints combined with fatigue, poor sleep, pain amplification, and other nonmusculoskeletal symptoms. The concept of fibromyalgia has clearly come a long way, but there are many miles to travel. The next two chapters will define fibromyalgia and describe those among us who are susceptible to it.

2
What Is Fibromyalgia?

A woman armed with sick headaches, nervousness, debility,
presentiments, fears, horrors, and all sorts of imaginary and
real diseases has an external armory of weapons of
subjugation.

Harriet Beecher Stowe (1811–1886),
Pink and White Tyranny, 1871

When the Arthritis Foundation tried to categorize the 150 different forms of musculoskeletal conditions in 1963, it created a classification known as *soft tissue rheumatism*. Included in this listing are conditions in which joints are *not* involved. Soft tissue rheumatism encompasses the supporting structures of joints (e.g., ligaments, bursae, and tendons), muscles, and other soft tissues. Fibromyalgia is a form of soft tissue rheumatism. A combination of three terms—*fibro-* (from the Latin *fibra*, or fibrous tissue), *myo-* (the Greek prefix *myos*, for muscles), and *algia* (from the Greek *algos*, which denotes pain)—fibromyalgia replaces earlier names for the syndrome that are still used by doctors and other health professionals such as *myofibrositis, myofascitis, muscular rheumatism, fibrositis,* and *generalized musculoligamentous strain*. Fibromyalgia is *not* a form of arthritis, since it is not associated with joint inflammation.

THE AMERICAN COLLEGE OF RHEUMATOLOGY (ACR) FIBROMYALGIA CRITERIA

In the late 1980s, a Multicenter Criteria Committee under the direction of Dr. Frederick Wolfe at the University of Kansas was formed to define fibromyalgia. In their study, 293 patients with presumed fibromyalgia were compared with 265 patients who had other rheumatic diseases in 16 centers throughout North America. The groups were evaluated for a variety of symptoms, signs, and laboratory abnormalities in an effort to ascertain which factors were the most *sensitive* and *specific* for defining the disorder. In other words, the investigators wanted to identify the most frequently found features of fibromyalgia (sensitivity) that could help doctors differentiate it from other disorders (specificity). The list in Table 1 (illustrated in Fig. 3) was 88.4 percent sensitive and 81.1 percent specific in identifying fibromyalgia patients. As a result, these criteria were endorsed in

1990 by the American College of Rheumatology (ACR), the association to which nearly all 5000 rheumatologists in the United States and Canada belong.

Focusing in on Table 1 and Figure 3, fibromyalgia essentially is:

1. Widespread pain of at least 3 months' duration (this rules out viruses or traumatic insults which resolve on their own).
2. Pain in all four quadrants of the body (picture cutting the body into quarters, as in a pie): right side, left side, above the waist, below the waist.
3. Pain occurring in at least 11 of 18 specified "tender" points (as shown in the figure) with at least one point in each quadrant.
4. Pain defined, in this context, as discomfort when 8 pounds of pressure are applied to the tender point.

Tender points usually occur in a specific distribution. For instance, 8 of the 18 tender points are in the upper back and neck area, and only 2 are below the

Table 1. *The 1990 ACR Criteria for Fibromyalgia*

1. *History of widespread pain.*

Definition: Pain is considered widespread when all of the following are present: pain in the left side of the body, pain in the right side of the body, pain above the waist and pain above the waist. In addition, axial skeletal pain (cervical spine or anterior chest or thoracic spine or low back) must be present. In this definition shoulder and buttock pain is considered as pain for each involved side. " Low back" pain is considered lower segment pain.

2. *Pain in 11 of 18 tender point sites on digital palpation.*

Definition: Pain, on digital palpation, must be present in at least 11 of the following 18 tender point sites:

Occiput: bilateral, at the suboccipital muscle insertions.

Low cervical: bilateral, at the anterior aspects of the inter-transverse spaces at C5–C7.

Trapezius: bilateral, at the midpoint of the upper border.

Supraspinatus: bilateral, at origins, above the scapula spine near the medial border.

2nd rib: bilateral, at the second costochondral junctions, just lateral to the junctions on upper surfaces.

Lateral epicondyle: bilateral, 2 cm distal to the epicondyles.

Gluteal: bilateral, in upper outer quadrants of buttocks in anterior fold of muscle.

Greater trochanter: bilateral, posterior to the trochanteric prominence.

Knees: bilateral, at the medial fat pad proximal to the joint line.

For a tender point to be considered "positive" the subject must state that the palpation was painful. "Tender" is not to be considered painful.

Note: For classification purposes patients will be said to have fibromyalgia if both criteria are satisfied. Widespread pain must have been present for at least 3 months. The presence of a second clinical disorder does not exclude the diagnosis of fibromyalgia.

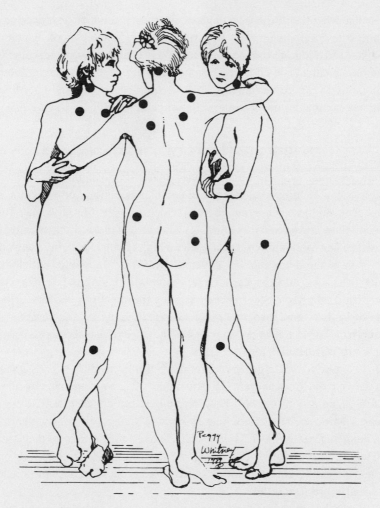

Fig. 3 *Fibromyalgia tender points. (Adapted from "The Three Graces,"*
Louvre Museum, Paris. From D. J. Wallace, The Lupus Book. *New York: Oxford*
University Press, 1995, p. 170; reprinted with permission from Dr. F. Wolfe.)

buttocks. The reader should be aware that tender points can occur almost anywhere in the body; the ACR criteria simply represent the most common 18
points. A consensus conference later agreed that the four factors listed above do
not have to be present at the same time in order to meet the criteria. Therefore, a
patient may have only right buttock pain on one day and left upper back pain on
another, or have different tender points on different days.

Once fibromyalgia was defined, it was possible to perform more reliable studies on this syndrome, since all researchers would be using the same definition.
We could now explore how many people in the United States had fibromyalgia,

determine what their primary complaints were, and identify groups of people on whom to test new treatments. Reporting a reproducible set of symptoms and signs has had additional fringe benefits: patients can be clearly educated on their condition; medical and other professional schools can teach students about fibromyalgia using a core terminology that has high sensitivity and specificity; and insurance companies now recognize fibromyalgia as a distinct syndrome.

OTHER FEATURES OF FIBROMYALGIA

In the previous chapter, we mentioned that fibromyalgia is associated with fatigue, sleep disturbances, and bowel complaints, among other symptoms and signs. How do these symptoms fit into the definition of fibromyalgia? The criteria committee considered these findings and correlated them statistically with the syndrome, but the symptoms did not have a high enough score in enough patients to be part of the definition. For example, Dr. Wolfe, in another article in 1990, stated that sleep disturbance, fatigue, numbness or tingling, and anxiety had more than a 60 percent occurrence in defining fibromyalgia, and headache or irritable bowel had more than a 50 percent occurrence. In fact, he observed that the presence of 7 of 18 tender points with 4 of the 6 features listed above was "highly suspicious" for the diagnosis.

In response to this, a group of international fibromyalgia experts issued what was termed the Copenhagen Declaration in 1992 and adopted by the World Health Organization in 1993. They recognized the use of the ACR criteria for research purposes but defined fibromyalgia as being part of a wider spectrum encompassing headache, irritable bladder, spastic colitis, painful menstrual periods, temperature sensitivity, atypical patterns of numbness and tingling, exercise intolerance, and complaints of weakness in addition to persistent fatigue, stiffness, and nonrestoring sleep.

It should be emphasized that disease definitions and criteria are always being updated and refined. In the next decade the ACR fibromyalgia criteria will probably be revised and hopefully will include newer forms of blood testing or brain imaging abnormalities.

FIBROMYALGIA TERMINOLOGY: CLASSIFICATION AND REGIONAL FORMS

Many rheumatologists recognize two types of fibromyalgia: primary and secondary. The cause of *primary fibromyalgia syndrome* is unknown, but it can be induced by trauma, infection, stress, inflammation, or other factors. *Secondary fibromyalgia* occurs when a primary condition, such as hypothyroidism or lupus, creates a concomitant fibromyalgia, the treatment of which may make the syndrome disappear. The next chapter will review this topic in more detail.

Sometimes, pain identical to that associated with fibromyalgia is located in specific areas or regions or in one quadrant of the body. For example, patients may have jaw and neck pain on one side and no discomfort anywhere else. Regional forms of fibromyalgia are called *regional myofascial syndrome* or *myofascial pain syndrome*. This entity is reviewed in detail in Chapter 12.

Finally, patients may hear a lot about trigger points or tender points. Many doctors consider them to be the same thing. However, for research purposes, there are subtle differences. A *tender point* is an area of tenderness in the muscles, tendons, bony prominences, or fat pads, whereas a *trigger point* shoots down to another area. For instance, when a trigger point is touched, it shoots pain to other muscles. Like pulling a trigger in a gun, it sends out a bullet that travels, and pain can be felt in areas away from the trigger.

SUMMING UP

The term *fibromyalgia* refers to a complex syndrome characterized by pain amplification, musculoskeletal discomfort, and systemic symptoms. Although its existence was questioned in the past, nearly all rheumatologists, medical societies, and the overwhelming majority of physicians now accept fibromyalgia as a distinct diagnostic entity.

3
Who Gets Fibromyalgia and Why?

*I am glad my case is not serious but these nervous troubles
are dreadfully depressing.*
                    Charlotte Perkins Gilman (1860–1935),
                            The Yellow Wallpaper, 1913

When fibromyalgia is first diagnosed, patients often have two reactions. The first reaction is relief. They have a legitimate diagnosis and are not crazy. Then a feeling of loneliness and a hint of fear can be detected, since most patients have never heard of the fibromyalgia syndrome and do not know what to do. It is worth repeating that the intent of this book is to promote a better understanding of fibromyalgia, as well as to provide patients, allied health professionals, and physicians with ways to work together. But first, this chapter will discuss how many people have fibromyalgia and how it might have been acquired.

HOW PREVALENT IS FIBROMYALGIA?

Until recently, nobody knew how many people had fibromyalgia. Dr. Frederick Wolfe, the same physician who chaired the ACR Criteria Committee, received funding to undertake an epidemiologic survey of the syndrome. Using computerized applications of field methodologies to estimate the prevalence of fibromyalgia (the number of cases per 100,000 individuals), his team estimated that 6 million people in the United States fulfill the ACR criteria for fibromyalgia. This and other surveys suggest that while 2 percent of the adult U.S. population have full-blown fibromyalgia (3.5 percent of adult women and 0.5 percent of adult men), 11 percent have chronic widespread pain and 20 percent have chronic regional pain.

Fibromyalgia is the third or fourth most common reason for consulting a rheumatologist. Approximately 15–20 percent of all patients seeking rheumatology referrals have fibromyalgia. The 5000 rheumatologists in the United States who are trained in internal medicine and subspecialize in managing more than 150 musculoskeletal and immune system disorders are very familiar with the diagnosis and treatment of fibromyalgia.

WHO DEVELOPS FIBROMYALGIA?

Even though 1 American in 50 has fibromyalgia, the syndrome is distributed unevenly across the population. For reasons that are not known, 80–90 percent of patients with the disorder are women. (One theory contends that women have a lower pain threshold than men, which is hormonally related.) Fibromyalgia is extremely uncommon in children and rarely appears for the first time in older persons. Within these groups, complaints and clinical features are atypical (see Chapter 16). In the United States, fibromyalgia is more common among Caucasians than among other racial groups. Using the ACR criteria or other earlier suggested criteria, the prevalence of fibromyalgia in other countries or regions (mostly in Europe, Canada, and Australia) has ranged from 0.5 percent to 12 percent. Some researchers have observed an increased prevalence among first-generation immigrant families in the United States. For instance, our research group has been struck by the relatively high prevalence of fibromyalgia among newly arrived Iranians and Russians.

Are humans the only species to develop fibromyalgia? Probably not. Lameness has been observed in dogs for some time, and articles in the veterinary literature convincingly show that they can also have tender points.

HOW OLD DO YOU HAVE TO BE TO GET FIBROMYALGIA?

Most of our fibromyalgia patients are in their prime of life and at the peak of their careers. Surveys have shown that most patients develop the syndrome in their 30s and 40s. Fibromyalgia infrequently evolves during adolescence. Whereas 60 percent of cases are diagnosed in people between the ages of 30 and 49, another 35 percent of patients are diagnosed in their 20s or between the age of 50 and 65. The reasons for this distribution are not clear, but the decline in onset after the age of 50 may have something to do with menopause in women, which may alleviate (but occasionally aggravate) certain fibromyalgia symptoms.

IS FIBROMYALGIA GENETIC?

In the mid-1980s, one research study suggested that fibromyalgia patients had an increased prevalence of a specific gene. These results, however, were shown to be inaccurate when confirmatory studies were performed on a larger scale. Even though no fibromyalgia genetic markers have been found, we are aware of studies documenting a high prevalence of the syndrome among certain families. Whether this is due to a yet-undiscovered genetic marker or markers, or from environmental or psychological factors is still unclear. Recently, Dr. Yunus has conducted studies suggesting that pain amplification may be genetically mediated.

WHAT ARE SOME OF THE CAUSES OF FIBROMYALGIA?

What turns on the fibromyalgia syndrome? The biology, chemistry, hormonal factors, and immune factors involved are detailed in Part II of this book. However, when we ask patients what they feel caused their fibromyalgia, trauma, infections, and stress are the three most common responses.

Fibromyalgia resulting from a single-event trauma

Becky was enjoying the feel of her brand-new roadster when somebody who wasn't paying attention rear-ended her at 10 miles per hour while she was stopped at a red light. The bumper was dented, and so was Becky's future. A day later, she began to complain of stiffness and aching in her upper back and neck, along with headaches. She was initially diagnosed on the basis of a stiff neck as having a whiplash injury. Dr. Allen treated her with ibuprofen, a soft neck collar, and a mild muscle relaxant. When she failed to improve, physical therapy was prescribed a week later. Over the next 3 months, Becky's pain spread to her lower back, legs, and elbows. She could no longer sleep through the night. The pain worsened as the day progressed or if the weather changed. Her skin became sensitive to the touch, particularly if the physical therapist worked her too hard. Dr. Allen diagnosed her as having post-traumatic fibromyalgia and initiated a specific treatment program.

When we last counted, there were 47 different reported secondary causes of fibromyalgia. *According to patients*, the most common cause of secondary fibromyalgia is trauma. There are two types of trauma: injury resulting from a single event or continuous trauma with resulting repetitive injury.

First, let's discuss a single-event injury. Suppose that in your community 100 people sustain a whiplash injury from a 10-mile-per-hour rear-ender automobile accident on a given day. A whiplash injury occurs when a car driver or passenger is rear-ended. The head and neck stay still at first, while the body jerks forward. As the body returns back, the neck hyperextends backward. What happens to people after a whiplash injury? Many will go to their doctor within days and report pain in their upper back and neck areas. Their doctor will prescribe ibuprofen or naproxen-like anti-inflammatory agents, a muscle relaxant, and perhaps even a small prescription for a strong pain killer. A minority may be given a neck collar or physical or chiropractic therapy. After 2–3 months, all but 2–5 percent (up to 21 percent in some studies) of the patients will get better and gradually discontinue all therapy. But what about the remaining people? Strange things start to happen. For completely unclear reasons, these 2–5 percent begin to hurt more and their pain becomes widespread. They complain of lower back and leg pain (areas that were not injured), begin noticing difficulty sleeping, and become fatigued. Ultimately, they are diagnosed as having fibromyalgia. Many doctors don't understand this; they suffered the same trivial injury with the same impact from which other patients fully recover! We have seen this with slip-and-fall injuries and other forms of minor trauma. This phenomenon is poorly documented in the medical literature, and since litigation frequently is involved, many doctors are not very sympathetic and suspect the wish for secondary gain. Some insurance companies have taken the position that posttraumatic fibromyalgia does not exist. Case reports in the literature are not enough, although the scenario involving Becky has recently been validated by Dr. Wolfe's group in a scientifically acceptable manner. We have seen it happen hundreds of times, even when no lawsuit is in the offing, but we do not know why.

Fibromyalgia from continuous trauma

Although Jared was found to have scoliosis as a child, it did not interfere with his activities or lifestyle. After graduating from junior college, he took a job as a shipping clerk. His responsibilities included preparing packages for delivery that weighed up to 50 pounds and carrying them to the loading dock. Jared also had to log the shipment's specifications onto the company's computer and track when they were sent and received. After 6 weeks on the job, Jared started to notice discomfort in his upper and lower back and experienced occasional numbness in his left hand. At first, naproxen (Aleve) relieved the symptoms, and he noted that the pain diminished on weekends. After 3 months on the job, Jared was barely able to make it to work. A family physician gave him a muscle relaxant and a few hydrocodone bitartrate/acetaminophen (Vicodin) to take for severe pain and prescribed physical therapy. He felt better after the therapy sessions, but relief did not last. His family physician referred Jared to an orthopedist, who requested an occupational therapy evaluation. Ginger, the therapist, closely scrutinized how Jared lifted boxes and supported his weight in relation to his scoliosis and the company's holding tables. She also watched how Jared sat and functioned when he worked at the computer. Ginger recommended that he wear a lumbar band at work, taught him how to straddle his weight, and adjusted the height and back of the computer chair. Jared was instructed in strengthening exercises, and the computer monitor's angle was altered. Jared now takes only Aleve occasionally and is largely pain free.

Jared's complaints are extremely common. Repetitive trauma from poor workstation body mechanics (usually associated with regional myofascial syndrome) is especially common among workers who do heavy lifting. The legal term "continuous trauma" opens up another can of worms because it also involves litigation, particularly worker's compensation. Chapters 12 and 24 discuss repetitive strain syndrome and disability issues in more detail.

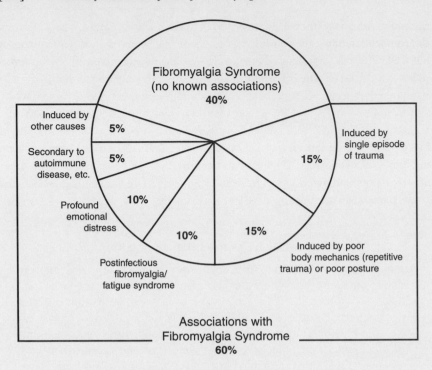

Fig. 4 *Distribution of fibromyalgia syndrome in the United States.*

What about infections?

One of the most common self-reported causes of fibromyalgia is an infectious process, possibly a viral (e.g., an Epstein-Barr-like) illness characterized by fever, swollen glands, sore throat, and cough. When these conditions disappear, the patient develops profound aching and fatigue. Over 40 microbes have been associated with postinfectious fatigue syndromes and are reviewed in Chapter 13. The inciting organisms are quite diverse and include parvovirus, the herpes virus causing mononucleosis and Epstein-Barr, *Toxoplasma gondii*, hepatitis A virus, cytomegalovirus, *Brucella*, poliovirus, the virus causing AIDS, and the bacterium causing Lyme disease.

Can emotional stress cause fibromyalgia?

Severe emotional stress or trauma frequently triggers and aggravates fibromyalgia. Psychologists have devised an inventory that they call a "Life Events Questionnaire." Bad things that can happen to people are rated numerically on the basis of severity. For example, the death of a child or spouse is more traumatic than losing a job or simply having a bad day. There is little doubt that fibromyalgia can come about or be accelerated by a diminished ability to cope with life's stresses and traumas. How does this happen? Part II of this book will survey models of stress that have been studied with regard to our hypothalamic-pituitary-adrenal (or stress hormone) axis and how this relates to fibromyalgia.

Associations with primary fibromyalgia

Forty percent of fibromyalgia cases appear spontaneously, and no obvious inciting factor is ever found. This condition is termed *primary fibromyalgia syndrome*. It is united by core features (widespread musculoskeletal pain and tender points), characteristic features (fatigue, stiffness, sleep disorder), and associated features (anxiety, depression, numbness, irritable bowel), and no specific inciting event is associated with its onset.

Other associations with fibromyalgia

Other triggers of fibromyalgia include autoimmune diseases, withdrawal from medications (especially steroids), prescription of other medications (such as interferons), and hormonal abnormalities (particularly low thyroid level). Figure 4 shows some of the associations with fibromyalgia.

The next (and most complex) part of this book reviews the basic science of fibromyalgia.

Part II
BASIC SCIENCE AND FIBROMYALGIA

Pain is perfect misery, the worst of evils and excessive, overturns all patience.

John Milton (1608–1674),
Paradise Lost, 1667

The next four chapters discuss what makes fibromyalgia a *pain amplification syndrome*. We will first review the path normal pain takes and then relate why things might go awry in fibromyalgia. There are many candidates whose potential deviousness will be evaluated. Abnormal connections between hormones, the immune system, sleep physiology, muscle pathology, and abnormalities of the nervous system are described. Unlike the rest of the book, this part uses a lot of technical language. Table 2 and the Glossary will help the reader navigate Part II successfully. You may wish to skip this part at this time and return to it later.

4

Why and How Do We Hurt?

*When pain is unbearable it destroys us; when it does not it is
bearable.*
> Marcus Aurelius (121–180), *Meditations vi*, c. 170 A.D.

A fibromyalgia patient frequently complains of pain. The pain of fibromyalgia is
different from that of a headache, stomach cramp, toothache, or swollen joint. It
has been described as a type of stiffness or aching, often associated with spasm.
Unlike the other pains mentioned above, fibromyalgia pain responds poorly to
aspirin, acetaminophen (Tylenol), or ibuprofen (Advil, Motrin). In fact, studies
have suggested that even narcotics such as morphine are minimally beneficial in
ameliorating fibromyalgia pain. Why is it that fibromyalgia patients can take
codeine, Darvon, Vicodin, or even Demerol for musculoskeletal aches and have
only a slight response?

In this chapter, we'll explore what makes fibromyalgia a pain amplification
syndrome. Why does the patient hurt in places where there was often no injury
and all laboratory tests are normal? What creates what doctors call *allodynia*, or a
clinical situation that results in pain from a stimulus (such as light touch) that normally should *not* be painful? Fibromyalgia is a form of chronic, widespread allodynia, as well as sustained *hyperalgesia*, or greater sensitivity than would be
expected to an adverse stimulus.

NORMAL PAIN PATHWAYS

The nervous system consists of several components. The brain and spinal cord
comprise the *central nervous system*. Nerves leaving the spinal cord that tell us to
move our arms or legs are part of the "motor" aspects of the *peripheral nervous
system*. Additionally, all sorts of information about touch, taste, chemicals, and
pressure are relayed through "sensory" pathways back to the spinal cord, where
they are processed and sent up to the brain for a response. The *autonomic nervous
system* consists of specialized peripheral nerves.

ACUTE VERSUS CHRONIC PAIN

Fibromyalgia is a disorder characterized by an inappropriate neuromuscular reaction that leads to chronic pain. Patients with fibromyalgia usually react

normally to acute pain. Our current concepts of the way the body responds to chronic painful stimuli stem from the *gate theory*, first proposed by Melzack and Wall in 1965. Nerve "wires" go from the periphery to the dorsal horn of the spinal cord. These wires are modulated by feedback loops within the nervous system. Each wire ending, or "gate," may open or close in response to pain impulses. Structures in the lower part of the brain known as the *brain stem* receive notice of this input at the spinal cord level and signal it how to respond.

To elaborate upon this, nerve wires from the skin, muscles, or joints send sensory signals (e.g., touch, pressure) to the spinal cord. Several separate sensory pathways have been described. The particular sensory trail important in fibromyalgia is one termed *nociception*. A *nociceptor* is a receptor that is sensitive to a noxious stimulus. Nociceptors are present in blood vessel walls, muscle, fascia, tendons, joint capsules, fat pads, and on body surfaces. A noxious stimulus can be thermal (heat, cold), mechanical (touch, pressure), or chemical. Normally, the body transmits these nociceptive impulses neurochemically from the periphery to the central nervous system. *One factor that distinguishes acute from chronic pain is that the perception of chronic pain is significantly influenced by the interaction of physiologic, psychological, and social processes.* Unlike patients with acute pain, those with chronic pain often don't appear to be in pain.

Types of wiring and insulation

All sorts of fibers make up the wires that connect the periphery to the spinal cord. Some of the wires are quite heavy and insulated, while others are thin and unprotected. The nociceptive pathway is transmitted to the spinal cord by *unmyelinated* (uninsulated) *C fibers* and *myelinated* (insulated) *A-delta (Group 3)* fibers (Fig. 5). For example, unmyelinated C fibers carry diffuse, burning pain sensations, while myelinated A-delta fibers transmit signals from strong, noxious stimuli potentially damaging to tissues. *B fibers* are myelinated nerves that are part of the autonomic nervous system. In a part of the spinal cord known as the *dorsal root ganglion*, a group of chemicals known as *neuropeptides* are released and travel up to the brain. Neuropeptides transmit nociceptive signals to spinal cord nerve cells and modulate (amplify or downgrade) the body's pain response. They have exotic names that only a neurophysiologist could be proud of, including, among others, *substance P, calcitonin-related gene peptide, norepinephrine, enkephalin-containing interneurons,* and *neurokinin A.* From the dorsal horn of the spinal cord, neuropeptides transmit information about the intensity and quality of the signal from the spine up to the thalamus of the brain via the *spinothalamic tract.* The thalamus interprets sensory and discriminative aspects of pain and sends messages further up the brain, which processes these signals and secretes a chemical known as *endorphin*, which can mute or eliminate pain. The brain sends signals back down the spinal cord via *adrenalin* (epinephrine)

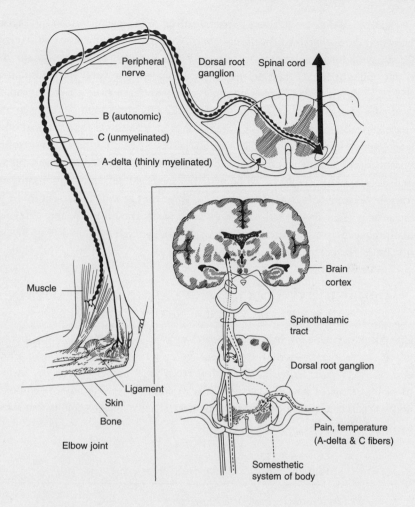

Fig. 5 *Normal pain pathways. Signals from pain receptors in muscles, joints, skin, ligaments, and bone are transmitted by A-delta and C fibers to the spinal cord. A-delta and C signals are sent to the thalamus of the brain via the spinothalamic tract after exiting the dorsal root ganglion, where neurotransmitters are released.*

and *serotonin,* the principal neurotransmitters of the descending system. Serotonin is a remarkable chemical that we will talk more about later. In addition to nociception, serotonin is capable of regulating mood, arousal, aggression, sleep, learning, nerve growth, and appetite.

Before we complete the cast of characters, there are a few other bit players that have a role in our pain production team. Certain chemicals are *proinflammatory,* or capable of inducing inflammation. These include certain types of *prostaglandins* and *bradykinins.*

Finally, it's time to introduce a special subset of the peripheral nervous system, known as the *autonomic nervous system* (*ANS*). The ANS consists of two types of fibers: sympathetic and parasympathetic. The *sympathetic nervous system* (*SNS*) is our "fight or flight" mechanism. It releases adrenalin when we are threatened and "revs up the juices," resulting in aggressive behavior or self-protection. The ANS also regulates our pulse and blood pressure by constricting or dilating blood vessels. Additionally, the ANS can relax or contract muscles and regulate sweat, urine, and defecation reflexes. The ability of the SNS to stimulate sensory fibers that meld into the nociceptive pathway is extremely important. At the same time that nociceptive influences are being processed and sent up the spinothalamic tract, parallel signals from B (autonomic) fibers are received and sent to the limbic system of the brain via the *spinoreticular tract*. The limbic system helps modulate many of our emotions, including alertness, vigilance, and fear. Figure 5 illustrates normal nociceptive processes.

ORGANIC PAIN: LOCALIZED VERSUS CENTRAL PAIN; NOCICEPTIVE VERSUS NEUROPATHIC PAIN

Chronic pain can be *organic* (real) or *psychogenic*, where patients think their pain is physical. Organic sources of pain can be either *peripheral* or *central*. Peripheral pain results in muscular discomfort from local tender points. For instance, local injections of anesthetics such as novocaine or xylocaine can temporarily abolish pain at a specific site. Exercising a muscle can lead to pain in that muscle, as shown in Figure 6.

Table 2. *Pain Classifications Relevant to Fibromyalgia*

  I. Acute pain—usually reacts normally in fibromyalgia
 II. Chronic pain
   A. Psychogenic pain—not part of fibromyalgia
   B. Organic pain
     1. Location
       a. Localized—observed in regional myofascial pain
       b. Central—observed in fibromyalgia
     2. Source
       a. Neuropathic—not part of fibromyalgia; due to damaged or injured nerves, as in diabetes, trauma, and herniated disc
       b. Nociceptive—includes features of fibromyalgia (see Glossary for definitions)
         (i) Hyperalgesia
         (ii) Neuroplasticity
         (iii) Causalgia
         (iv) Hyperpathia
       c. Non-nociceptive (allodynia)—can function as nociceptive fibers with chronic stimulation in fibromyalgia

---

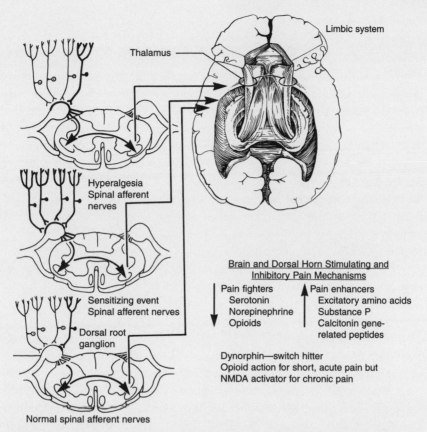

Limbic system

Thalamus

Hyperalgesia
Spinal afferent
nerves

Sensitizing event
Spinal afferent nerves

Dorsal root
ganglion

Normal spinal afferent nerves

Brain and Dorsal Horn Stimulating and
Inhibitory Pain Mechanisms

Pain fighters	Pain enhancers
Serotonin	Excitatory amino acids
Norepinephrine	Substance P
Opioids	Calcitonin gene-related peptides

Dynorphin—switch hitter
Opioid action for short, acute pain but
NMDA activator for chronic pain

Fig. 6 *Pain amplification in fibromyalgia. Chronic sensitization of A-delta and C pain fibers leading to the thalamus and B fibers leading to the limbic system alters the normal system of releasing chemicals that enhance or fight pain.*

On the other hand, pain can emanate from brain and spinal cord pathways without any peripheral tissue or nociceptive input or stimulus. A classical example is something doctors call *phantom limb* pain. Let us say that a patient has had a leg amputated below the left knee but complains that the left ankle hurts. This seems impossible, but it happens all the time. This is due to a phenomenon known as *neuroplasticity,* in which prolonged central stimulation without peripheral input and excitation of pain fibers creates a chronic pain sensation below the amputation site.

Finally, chronic organic pain is either *nociceptive*, as in fibromyalgia, non-nociceptive, or *neuropathic*. Nociceptive pain occurs with chronic, repeated stimulation and can potentially produce tissue damage. In this circumstance, non-nociceptive fibers can act as nociceptive ones. Neuropathic pain results from a direct nerve injury that leads to nervous system dysfunction. Examples of neuropathic pain include diabetes, trauma, and herniated disc. These concepts are summarized in Table 2.

WHAT GOES WRONG THAT MAKES FIBROMYALGIA PATIENTS HURT?

Hyperalgesia is an exaggerated response to a painful stimulus. Inappropriately increased hyperalgesia results when repeated stimuli from areas within tissues lower the thresholds for activating nociceptors. As a result, seemingly innocuous stimuli such as light touching can cause severe pain. For example, lack of oxygen to a capillary beneath the skin in the presence of a low pH (or acidic environment) is capable of activating, exciting, and sensitizing nociceptors. Another study has shown that fibromyalgia patients react to pain after stimulation with a carbon dioxide laser with greater nociceptive evoked electrical activity than do healthy people. These actions lead to perceptual amplification, or a state of hypervigilance.

The mechanism or mechanisms that cause(s) nociceptive pain loops to amplify pain rather than suppress pain in fibromyalgia is the subject of considerable debate. And as in any political debate, there are several candidates.

Candidate 1: Substance P

Substance P stands for pain. Consisting of 11 amino acids (building blocks of protein), it is a neurotransmitter released in the dorsal root ganglion of the spinal cord, which results in greater pain perception by promoting blood vessel dilation and extravasation (leakage) into the plasma of a host of irritants, proinflammatory chemicals, and white blood cells (Fig. 6). Blood levels of substance P are normal in fibromyalgia, but two research centers have shown that its levels are increased in the spinal fluid of fibromyalgia patients. Sustained activation of substance P along with neurokinins lowers the pain threshold. Therefore, agents that block substance P may help patients with fibromyalgia. An example of this is capsaicin, a topical salve consisting of the chemical used in cayenne pepper and sold commercially as Zostrix or Dolorac. Unfortunately, the story is not as clear-cut as we would like. For example, patients with more severe fibromyalgia tend to have lower substance P levels. Also, substance P is broken down by a chemical that is not present in the spinal cord, and substance P spinal fluid levels could thus be artificially elevated. Recently, Dr. Jon Russell, a rheumatologist at the University of Texas, San Antonio, found preliminary evidence that an increase in levels of nerve growth factor, a chemical that promotes substance P production, is also present in the spinal fluid of fibromyalgia patients.

Candidate 2: Serotonin

Serotonin regulates the brain's ability to control pain and modulates mood, motivation, and behavior. Serotonin is also the major descending neurotransmitter of nociceptive responses from the brain back to the spinal cord. Dr. Jon Russell has performed numerous studies suggesting that serotonin deficiency, both centrally and peripherally, is a key source of fibromyalgia pain and pathology. Serotonin is stored and released by platelets, cells that promote blood clotting. Normally, an amino acid known as *tryptophan* is metabolized to serotonin. For many years, L-tryptophan was available over the counter as a sleep aid. However, a contaminant in the manufacture of L-tryptophan produced a variant of the autoimmune disease scleroderma, and it was taken off the market in 1989. Unfortunately, in some patients, L-tryptophan travels via an alternate route, known as the *kynurenine pathway*, rather than via the serotonin pathway, which promotes anxiety and irritability. Russell's studies found decreased serum levels of serotonin, tryptophan, and other amino acids in the spinal fluid in fibromyalgia suggest or lead to a variety of effects. These include less hypothalamic-pituitary-adrenal (or hormone-stress) axis activity (see Chapter 6), poor sleep, increased pain perception, alterations in substance P, and lower levels of growth and sex hormones. However, this hypothesis, although attractive, does not answer many questions. For instance, drugs that promote serotonin activity by themselves have little impact on the disease, and patients with degenerative osteoarthritis have lower serotonin levels than those with fibromyalgia.

Candidate 3: Excitatory amino acids

As discussed, Dr. Russell and others found that a group of amino acids in addition to tryptophan are decreased in the spinal fluid of fibromyalgia patients. Stimulated, unmyelinated C fibers promote the release of these amino acids and activate a receptor known as *N*-methyl-D-aspartic acid (NMDA), which produces painful signals (see Fig. 6). These receptors are activated in chronic pain but not in acute pain. Fibromyalgia is perpetuated when neurokinin and NMDA receptors remain activated and produce a sustained hyperexcitability state. An anesthetic known as *ketamine* selectively blocks NMDA receptors and produces the most dramatic fibromyalgia pain relief ever reported. Another anesthetic may also play a role, but the pain produced by NMDA receptors is not blocked by opioids (morphine derivatives). Substance P and the amino acid L-arginine promote the release of nitric oxide, which is also a potent blood vessel dilator. Agents that block nitric oxide block the activity of NMDA receptors. Excitatory amino acids are the focus of intense scrutiny at this time.

Candidate 4: Opiates and endorphins

Enkephalins and endorphins are the body's natural opiates. These peptides (compounds with at least two amino acids) are parts of proteins. An *opiate* is a narcotic whose receptors play a role in chemical recognition and also have biologic actions. Endorphins are found in nerve cell membranes and are biologically active neuropeptides. Their blood and spinal fluid levels are normal in fibromyalgia. In addition to producing euphoria via the sympathetic nervous system's connections to the limbic system, opiates can interact with serotonin to decrease pain perception. The administration of morphine near the spinal cord modestly decreases pain levels in fibromyalgia. *Tricyclic* antidepressants such as amitriptyline (Elavil), the drugs most commonly used to treat fibromyalgia, promote the release of endorphin, which may account for some of their efficacy. Another opioid, *dynorphin*, also decreases acute pain but in chronic pain it becomes a "switch hitter," activating NMDA receptors and making chronic pain worse. We still know very little about this opiate.

What candidates are left? Can psychological and sociological factors affect pain perception?

Other chemicals that can produce pain in fibromyalgia are being studied. Some of them include prostaglandin products, calcitonin gene-related peptide (CGRP), and the cancer gene *c-fos*.

Finally, factors governing psychological behavior such as personality, mood, and attitude, as well as sociological factors such as work, economic status, culture, and family relationships can modify pain biologically by interacting with neuropeptides to alter pain perception. Chronic long-term pain, in turn, leads to decreased self-esteem and a reduced feeling of personal control. Figure 6 illustrates some of these interactions.

We have little doubt that other candidates will be nominated in the next few years.

SUMMING UP

Patients with fibromyalgia hurt when and where they should not. Pain amplification could be the result of "cross-circuiting" of neurotransmitters where the sustained release of certain chemicals results in more pain. Some of the possible disruptions in pain circuitry have been reviewed, but we know relatively little about what really goes on.

5

What's Wrong with My Muscles?

*The human body . . . indeed is like a ship; its bones being the
stiff standing-rigging, and the sinews the small running ropes,
that manage all the motions.*

Herman Melville (1819–1891)

Since most fibromyalgia patients complain of aching and spasm in their muscles,
common sense suggests that there must be something wrong with the muscle.
This is easier said than agreed upon. For the last 80 years, researchers have been
looking for the key to muscle pathology in fibromyalgia. As of this writing, there
are highly respected investigators who feel that there is little if anything wrong
with fibromyalgia muscles. However, other equally regarded researchers have
presented evidence that abnormal muscle metabolism is the linchpin for what
goes awry in the disorder.

Why are there such discrepancies? Let's explore what goes on in our muscles.

IS THERE ANYTHING WRONG WITH
MUSCLE STRUCTURE IN FIBROMYALGIA?

Our body has 640 different muscles, which constitute as much as 40 percent of
our weight. When physicians look at muscles of fibromyalgia patients under a
simple microscope, they generally appear normal. In fact, muscles must be
looked at under an electron microscope (which magnifies the tissue thousands of
times) in order to find any consistent abnormalities. In this setting there are subtle alterations, including the deposition of a chemical, glycogen, swollen and
abnormal cell organelles known as mitochondria, increased DNA fragmentation,
and smeared muscle cell membranes. Some investigators have shown that magnesium levels are low in the muscles of fibromyalgia patients. So where are the
disagreements? Fibromyalgia patients are generally deconditioned. In other
words, they are out of shape. Of course, many more people are out of shape than
have fibromyalgia, but studies of muscles from out-of-shape people also show
some of these alterations.

WHAT ABOUT MUSCLE FUNCTION?

If fibromyalgia muscles don't look very different from normal muscles under the
microscope, where else can we look for muscle pathology? Muscle strength can

be decreased or normal in fibromyalgia, and published studies conflict as to whether or not muscle fatigue is present. Nevertheless, people who are out of shape also have decreased muscle strength.

Let's look at blood flow to muscles. Muscles are fueled by oxygen, which is supplied and carried by arteries. Some muscles in fibromyalgia do not get enough oxygen. "Angina" of the muscles can develop, producing pain if the oxygen supply is decreased. (The heart is a muscle. Angina is cardiac chest pain brought on when not enough blood is supplied to the heart muscle via the coronary arteries.) Individuals who don't exercise regularly also have low tissue oxygenation. However, out-of-shape people don't necessarily have all the features reported in the *microcirculation* (small arteries and capillaries) of fibromyalgia patients. The diminished oxygen supply may also have to do with interactions between the ANS and the muscle in fibromyalgia. Other investigators minimize the role of the ANS and have performed experiments suggesting that the shape of red blood cell membranes is altered in fibromyalgia. This could adversely influence blood flow in small capillaries and prevent oxygen from reaching muscles and other tissues.

The body's immediate energy fuel is adenosine triphosphate (ATP). An enzyme involved in the production of ATP in muscles may be defective in fibromyalgia. Muscles become slower to consume glucose to produce energy, which diminishes energy reserves. When this happens, fibromyalgia patients don't utilize enough oxygen to meet their energy needs. Additionally, several researchers have examined the biochemistry of muscles by using a magnetic spectroscope not too different from the technology used in magnetic resonance imaging (MRI) scanning. A spectroscope is an instrument that analyzes light waves emitted by tissues. Some investigators report that fibromyalgia muscles have lower than normal levels of high-energy phosphates, but others counter that this condition is also seen in deconditioning.

Electrical activity in muscles can be assessed by an electromyogram (EMG). This "cardiogram of the muscles" also is normal when performed conventionally. However, if the EMG is performed with special maneuvers not usually performed with standard testing, fibromyalgic muscles may have difficulty relaxing after exertion and, when they are deprived of oxygen, have more spontaneous electrical activity.

THE BOTTOM LINE: MICROTRAUMA AND "TAUT BANDS" ARE PROBABLY RESPONSIBLE FOR MOST OF WHAT GOES WRONG WITH MUSCLES IN FIBROMYALGIA

Among others, Soren Jacobsen in Sweden and Robert Bennett at the University of Oregon put together concepts that might best explain what occurs in fibromyalgic muscles, developing what is known as the *microtrauma* or *taut band* hypothesis.

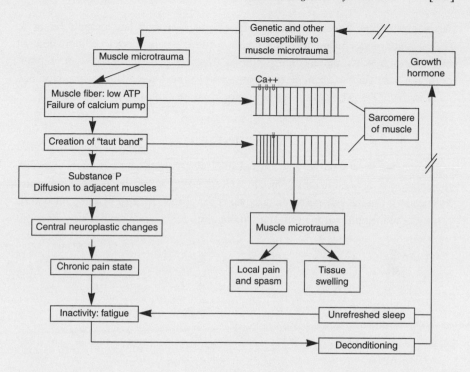

Fig. 7 *The muscle in fibromyalgia. Microtrauma creates a sequence of events leading to muscle spasm and not enough oxygen getting to muscles, which produces pain.*

Although unproven, it makes a lot of sense and represents a reasonable explanation worthy of the reader's time and effort to understand.

When healthy but sedentary people exert themselves abnormally, such as on a ski or hiking trip, this unaccustomed exertion results in muscle soreness and stiffness. Some of this pain could be due to microscopic muscle tears resulting in leakage of chemicals that produce discomfort. This usually lasts a day or two, and then the body's repair mechanisms take care of the problem. In fibromyalgia, the soreness and stiffness become chronic. How does this happen? Follow the sequences illustrated in Figure 7 as we describe this hypothesis.

When a focal injury affects a muscle fiber, it contains both relaxed and contracted units, or sarcomeres. This causes potassium to leave muscles and sarcomeres to stimulate Type C unmyelinated pain nerve endings. In turn, a calcium-ATP (or energy) pump is activated, unleashing events that produce a *taut band*. In other words, some of the muscle becomes as tight as a rubber band, while adjacent muscle relaxes. As a result of this chain of events, insufficient oxygen reaches muscles. Additionally, there are focal decreases in critical muscle enzyme levels that provide energy and fuel, as well as the release of substance P to nearby sarcomeres, producing pain and spasm. Some of these chemicals sensitize the nervous system, which perpetuates the vicious cycle of pain and spasm.

Also, growth hormone and its liver by-product, insulin-like growth factor 1 (IGF-1), are made during deep sleep and promote repair of muscles damaged by microtrauma. When patients sleep poorly, this repair is interfered with. Tender points occur at muscle-tendon junctions, where mechanical forces produce the most injury. This is discussed further in the next chapter.

SUMMING UP

Although muscles usually look normal in fibromyalgia, and although many of the changes described in muscle tissues reflect being out of shape, there are probably certain unique self-perpetuating events that produce muscle pain and spasm through the interplay of microtrauma, pain, chemicals, and unrefreshing sleep.

6

How Do Stress, Sleep, Hormones, and the Immune System Interact and Relate to Fibromyalgia?

*Canst thou not minister to a mind diseased / Pluck from
the memory a rooted sorrow / Raze out the written troubles of
the brain / And with some sweet oblivious antidote /
Cleanse the stuffed bosom of that perilous stuff / Which
weighs upon the heart?*
                William Shakespeare (1564–1616), *Macbeth*, 5:3–40

In medical school, students learn about the human body by *organ system*. They spend a few weeks on the heart, then the lung, followed by the gastrointestinal tract. Eventually the whole body is covered. One of the fascinating developments in the last decade has been the functional linkage and new connections of seemingly diverse body systems. Fibromyalgia research finally hit its stride when important studies connected the nervous system, the endocrine (hormone) system, and the immune system. This enabled physicians to devise improved strategies to help fibromyalgia patients. Basic background information provided in this chapter will be expanded upon in later parts of the book when we review treatments.

THE "STRESS HORMONE," OR HYPOTHALAMIC-PITUITARY-ADRENAL AXIS

Within the brain is a small region known as the *hypothalamus*. It makes releasing hormones that travel down a short path to the pituitary gland, which makes stimulating hormones. The stimulating hormones send signals to tissues where hormones are manufactured for specialized functions. Table 3 and Figure 8 show how thyroid, cortisol, insulin, breast milk, and growth hormone, are made along the hypothalamic-pituitary axis and the hypothalamic-pituitary-adrenal (HPA) axis.

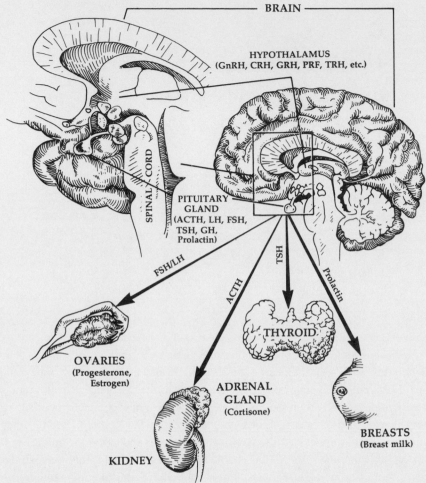

Fig. 8 *Hypothalamic and pituitary hormonal pathways. (From D. J. Wallace,* The Lupus Book. *New York: Oxford University Press, 1995, p. 123; reprinted with permission.)*

STRESS AND THE HPA AXIS

We have already mentioned that emotional stress can bring on or aggravate fibromyalgia. At the National Institutes of Health and the University of Michigan, studies have firmly established some of the factors important in this relationship. The role of corticotropin-releasing hormone (CRH), the precursor or ancestor of the steroid known as *cortisone*, has been the focus of much of this work. Even though CRH levels are normal in fibromyalgia, CRH responses (stress responses) to different forms of stimulation are blunted. CRH has many important interactions other than leading to the production of steroids. Its expression can be increased by stress, serotonin, and estrogen. Endorphins promote the

Table 3. *Important hormones derived from the hypothalamic-pituitary axis*

Hypothalamus (Releasers)	Pituitary (Stimulators)	Peripheral tissues (Hormones)
Corticotropin-releasing hormone	Adrenocorticotropic hormone	Cortisone
Thyrotropin-releasing hormone	Thyroid-stimulating hormone	Thyroid
Growth hormone–releasing hormone	Growth hormone	
Prolactin-releasing factor	Prolactin	Breast milk
Gonadotropin-releasing hormone	Follicle-stimulating hormone, luteinizing hormone	Estrogen, progesterone

secretion of CRH. Decreased sympathetic nervous system activity in the adrenal glands and substance P, as well as nitric oxide, can turn off CRH production. Rats with abnormally low stress responses develop many of the features we associate with fibromyalgia.

How do these interrelationships translate into a fibromyalgia patient's feeling of being unwell? The answer is not clear. However, these studies suggest that fibromyalgia patients do not respond normally to acute stress and do not release enough adrenalin. This leads to a chronic stress state to which the body reacts by making things worse, creating a vicious cycle that perpetuates the unwell feeling.

SLEEP AND FIBROMYALGIA

The average, healthy, well-adjusted adult gets up at seven-thirty in the morning feeling just terrible.

Jean Kerr (1923–)

Somewhere between 60 and 90 percent of fibromyalgia patients have difficulty sleeping. They might be in bed for 8 hours but do not wake up feeling refreshed, a condition termed *nonrestorative sleep*. Work done by Dr. Harvey Moldofsky at the University of Toronto since the 1970s has documented sleep brain wave abnormalities in fibromyalgia patients. If doctors attached an electroencephalograph (EEG) to the scalp and took a "cardiogram" of the brain of a sleeping healthy person, they would find four phases of sleep. Most of the time is taken up by a deep *slow wave sleep*, characterized by delta waves on the electrical tracing. Approximately 20 percent of sleep time is spent dreaming, which is termed *rapid eye movement* (REM) sleep. The majority of fibromyalgia patients have alpha

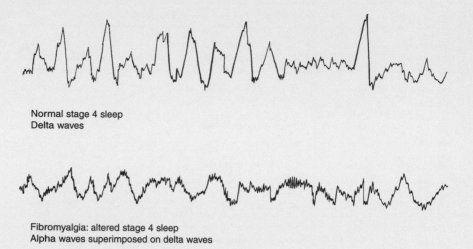

Normal stage 4 sleep
Delta waves

Fibromyalgia: altered stage 4 sleep
Alpha waves superimposed on delta waves

Fig. 9 *The alpha-delta sleep wave abnormality.*

waves (which should not be there) intruding into delta wave sleep, compared with only 10–15 percent of persons without the syndrome. Alpha-delta intrusion can have a startle effect and awaken the person. Sometimes, it may cause one to turn over, shake a leg, grit the teeth, or open the eyes. After a while, it keeps one from falling into a deep sleep. Some fibromyalgia patients have alpha-delta intrusion hundreds of times during an evening. It's no wonder that they wake up feeling more tired than before they went to sleep! Figure 9 illustrates alpha-delta sleep intrusion patterns in fibromyalgia patients.

HORMONES AND SLEEP

Even fully grown adults require growth hormone for a variety of purposes. Most growth hormone is produced when we are in slow (delta) wave sleep. Levels of a product of growth hormone known as *somatomedin C* are decreased by 30 percent in fibromyalgia, especially in the early morning. CRH also promotes the release of a chemical that blocks growth hormone secretion. Dr. Robert Bennett at the University of Oregon has theorized that the low levels of growth hormone observed in fibromyalgia patients (as measured by their by-products, IGF, or somatomedin C) make them more susceptible to muscle trauma because microtrauma occurring during the day cannot be repaired at night.

What does this mean in a practical sense? Abnormal electrical waves keep fibromyalgia patients up at night, which, in turn, prevents enough growth hormone from being made to repair and restore their muscles. Also, sleep can be augmented by the production of chemicals such as interleukin-1, tumor necrosis factor-alpha, acetylcholine, nitric oxide, and a hormone made by another part of the brain (pineal gland) known as *melatonin*. Moreover, fragmentation of sleep occurs with menstruation, stress, pain trauma, infection, or a change in the weather.

THE ROLE OF OTHER HORMONES IN FIBROMYALGIA

Additional hormones have been superficially studied in fibromyalgia. *Dehydroepiandrosterone (DHEA)*, an adrenal hormone, may be decreased in the syndrome. The *thyroid* hormone level is normal, but its responses to hypothalamic stimuli are blunted. A subset of fibromyalgia patients have elevated levels of *prolactin*, a hormone responsible for the secretion of breast milk, which may affect the immune system and muscles.

THE FINAL LINKAGE:
CONNECTING HORMONES AND NERVES WITH
THE IMMUNE SYSTEM AND CYTOKINES

What goes wrong with the immune system in fibromyalgia? When the body is attacked, the immune system comes to the rescue. We have a very sophisticated immune surveillance system, and it may come as a surprise that this system is reasonably intact in fibromyalgia. For example, in fibromyalgia studies of immune responsiveness, T-cell and B-cell counts, levels of autoantibodies (such as antinuclear antibody and rheumatoid factor), and the effectiveness of immunizations and allergy shots are usually normal. When I explain this to some patients, they ask why they develop so many infections or have lupus-like signs such as Raynaud's phenomenon (in which the fingers turn different colors in cold weather). There are explanations for this, some related to the ANS (see the next chapter) and others related to overlapping features with chronic fatigue syndrome (see Chapter 13).

One of the immune system's components involves a group of sugar-protein chemicals (or glycoproteins) known as *cytokines*. Cytokines play a role in the growth and development of T and B cells and have exotic names such as *interleukins* and *interferons*. They amplify or "gear up" T cells and B cells, which are types of white blood cells known as *lymphocytes*. Even though cytokine blood levels are normal in patients with fibromyalgia, the administration of cytokines to treat diseases (such as alpha-interferon to manage hepatitis or interleukin-2 for advanced cancer) *induces* or causes fibromyalgia. (Interleukin-6 also produces cognitive impairment.) As the first doctor to document this in the medical literature, I was amazed when my patients with advanced cancer at the City of Hope Medical Center developed fatigue, muscle aches, and difficulty connecting their thoughts within days of receiving interleukin-2. These fibromyalgia-like symp-

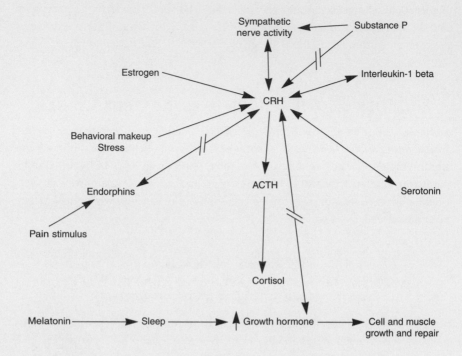

Fig. 10 *The body's "stress hormone" system. Cortisol, estrogen, pain chemicals, muscles, sleep, stress, and the ANS all interact with each other.*

toms lasted for several weeks and then disappeared even if no further therapy was given.

How does this relate to fibromyalgia? Dr. Jay Goldstein at the University of California, Irvine, has expanded upon these observations and developed the *limbic hypothesis* of fibromyalgia and fatigue syndromes. Since interleukin-1 beta can increase growth hormone, serotonin, ANS activity, endorphin, and CRH levels, as well as improve memory, sleep, and blood flow, Dr. Goldstein feels that the limbic area of the brain regulates these interactions. *Limbic encephalopathy*, or pathologic changes in the *limbic system* of the brain, could cause fibromyalgia, and chemicals that decrease the influence or effects of interleukin-1 beta worsen the syndrome.

Other complex interactions are also important. For instance, the cytokine tumor necrosis factor-alpha leads to the release of interleukin-1 beta, substance P, and interleukin-6, which aggravate fibromyalgia symptoms. Interleukin-2 levels can be increased by endorphins, which also promote T-cell proliferation. Substance P can stimulate T cells and cytokines. Interleukin-10 may improve fibromyalgia. Further, many interleukins have been shown to have brain receptors.

Figure 10 illustrates some of the disease interrelationships of hormones, sleep, and the immune system.

SUMMING UP

Certain hormone levels (especially CRH) are normal in fibromyalgia but respond sluggishly, especially to stress. Abnormal electrical brain waves interrupt normal sleep patterns, and this may influence normal responses of growth hormone, which, in turn, affects muscles. Administering cytokines can cause or improve fibromyalgia, and these chemicals are interconnected with hormonal and pain pathways.

We now are ready to add in another piece of this puzzle to what has already been introduced. Let's welcome the autonomic nervous system.

7

What Is the Autonomic Nervous System?

*Absence of psychoneurotic illness may be health
but it is not life.*
 D. W. Winnicott, *Playing with Reality*, 1971

The autonomic nervous system (ANS) has already been introduced; let's summarize what we know about it so far. Part of the peripheral nervous system, the ANS consists of the *sympathetic nervous system* (*SNS*), which consists of outflow from the thoracic and upper lumbar spine, and the *parasympathetic nervous system* (PNS), including outflow from the cranial nerves emanating from the upper spine and also from the mid-lumbar to the sacral areas at the buttock region. Several neurochemicals help transmit autonomic instructions. These include *epinephrine* (adrenalin), *norepinephrine* (noradrenalin), *dopamine*, and *acetylcholine*. This chapter will focus on how abnormalities in the regulation of the ANS cause many of the symptoms and signs observed in fibromyalgia.

THE WORKINGS OF THE ANS

Our body has numerous receptors or surveillance sensors that detect heat, cold, and inflammation. These ANS sensors perform a function known as *autoregulation*. As an example of how the ANS normally works, why don't we pass out when we suddenly jump out of bed? Because the ANS instantly constricts our blood vessels peripherally and dilates them centrally. In other words, as blood is pooled to the heart and the brain, the ANS adjusts our blood pressure and regulates our pulse, or heart rate, so that we don't collapse. On the local level, these sensors dilate or constrict flow from blood vessels. They can secondarily contract and relax muscles, open and close lung airways, or cause us to sweat. For instance, ANS sensors can tone muscles, regulate urine, and regulate bowel movements, as well as dilate or constrict our pupils. The SNS arm of the ANS is our "fight or flight" system, releasing epinephrine and norepinephrine as well as a neurochemical called *dopamine*. Whereas the SNS often acts as an acute stress response, the PNS arm tends to protect and conserve body processes and resources. The SNS and PNS sometimes work at cross purposes, but frequently

they work together to permit actions such as normal sexual functioning and urination (see Table 4a).

INTERACTIONS BETWEEN FIBROMYALGIA AND
AN ABNORMALLY REGULATED ANS

How do the workings of the ANS relate to fibromyalgia? The SNS is underactive
in fibromyalgia, which results in low blood flow rates, leaky capillaries, and a
relatively low blood pressure baseline. In the spinal fluid, norepinephrine and
neuropeptide Y (a neuropeptide similar to epinephrine which acts as a sensor for
the ANS, increases appetite, and calms nerves) levels are decreased. *Tilt-table
testing,* in which patients lay down and are tilted upward on an examining table,
shows normal baseline pulse and blood pressure but an exaggerated rise in blood
pressure in many fibromyalgia patients. Some fibromyalgia patients have *neurally mediated hypotension,* in which decreased sympathetic activity lowers
blood pressure, leading to dizziness and fatigue.

According to Dr. Daniel J. Clauw at Georgetown University, the ANS control
mechanisms are out of sync in certain patients with fibromyalgia. Sensors dilate
the blood vessels in one area and constrict them in an adjacent region without
reason or provocation. Termed *autonomic dysregulation,* or *dysautonomia,* this
loss of autoregulatory or local control causes a variety of clinical problems associated with fibromyalgia.

Table 4a. *Normal autonomic functions*

Area	Sympathetic nervous system	Parasympathetic nervous system
Neurotransmitter	Norepinephrine, epinephrine Acetylcholine, dopamine	Acetylcholine
Saliva	Increases	Increases
Tears	Decreases	Increases
Pupils	Dilates	Constricts
Heart	Increases contraction, blood pressure Dilates coronary arteries	Decreased contraction Constricts coronary arteries
Lungs	Opens up airways	Closes airways
Gi tract	Slows down peristalsis	Increases peristalsis
Sex	Allows male ejaculation	Allows male erection
Bladder	Contracts the bladder	Relaxes the bladder
Skin	Produces sweat Constricts blood vessels	—
Muscles	Constricts blood flow	—
Sweat	Increases	

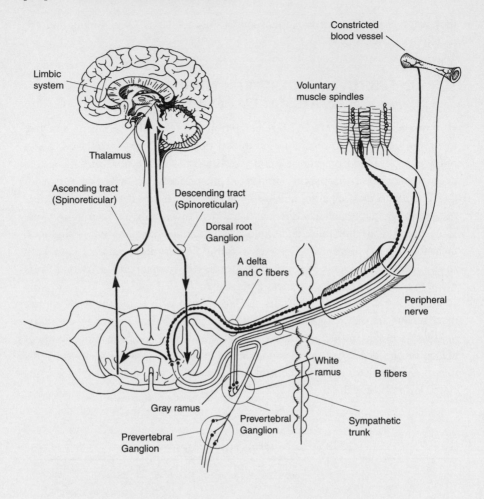

Fig. 11 *The ANS. Autonomic signals are carried by B fibers to the spinal cord and ascend to the limbic system of the brain via the spinoreticular tract.*

How do the ANS sensors lose their fine-tuning control? As discussed in Chapter 4 and shown in Fig. 11, autonomic signals are transmitted from the periphery by events such as physical trauma or changes in posture by myelinated B fibers via a few detours to the spinal cord. From there the ANS ascends the spinal cord via the spinoreticular tract to the limbic system of the brain. In fibromyalgia, however, repeated incoming signals from unmyelinated C fibers to the dorsal horn of the spinal cord may also create nociceptor hypersensitivity, overwhelming sympathetic controls and leading to blood vessel constriction and hyperalgesia. When this leads to the appearance or sensation of swelling, it is called *neurogenic inflammation*. Further, substance P can activate SNS receptors in the dorsal root ganglion. In other words, while SNS activity is decreased in fibromyalgia, the system itself is hypervigilant and probably overreacts to unimportant stimuli.

DYSAUTONOMIA ALLOWS FIBROMYALGIA TO MIMIC AUTOIMMUNE DISEASES

Altered SNS tone can mimic immunologic or autoimmune disorders. Autoimmune disorders occur when the body becomes allergic to itself. Dysautonomia produces *reactive hyperemia*, or redness in the skin after palpation. This leads to a mottled appearance under the skin and can mimic or cause *dermatographia* (rubbing a key into the skin produces an impression that lasts for minutes), *livedo reticularis* (a red, lace-like, checkerboard appearance under the skin), and *Raynaud's phenomenon*. All of these features, particularly Raynaud's phenomenon (which is what happens when your fingers become patriotic by turning red, white, and blue when exposed to cold temperatures), are prominent features of autoimmune diseases such as systemic lupus erythematosus and scleroderma, which are also characterized by dysautonomia and neurogenic inflammation. One of the procedures used to diagnose systemic lupus is the lupus band test. In the early 1980s, some investigators reported that this skin biopsy was giving false-positive readings in fibromyalgia patients. Occasional deposits of small amounts of immune complexes (which give the false-positive result) were shown to result from leaky capillaries observed with autonomic dysfunction. We have seen patients erroneously diagnosed with lupus who really had fibromyalgia with dysautonomia.

THE CLINICAL SPECTRUM OF FIBROMYALGIA RESULTING FROM DYSAUTONOMIA: HYPERVIGILANCE OF BODILY FUNCTIONS

Abnormal autonomic regulation leads to many secondary clinical syndromes that can be part of fibromyalgia or fall into the realm of *fibromyalgia-related conditions*. Most of these conditions are discussed in detail in Chapters 13 and 14 and are listed in Table 4b. They include mitral valve prolapse, noncardiac chest pain, migraine/tension headache syndrome, irritable bowel syndrome (also called *spastic colitis* or *functional bowel syndrome*), premenstrual syndrome, and female urethral syndrome (irritable bladder).

Infrequently, serious derangement of the ANS leads to prolonged stimulation of pain amplifiers, which results in chronic neurogenic inflammation. The most important complication of this is a condition of symapthetically mediated pain known as *reflex sympathetic dystrophy*, which is reviewed in Chapter 13.

The hypervigilance associated with dysautonomia results in fibromyalgia

Table 4b. *Examples of autonomic dysfunction in fibromyalgia*

Neurally mediated hypotension—abnormally low blood pressure

Mitral valve prolapse—causes palpitations due to release of epinephrine, which increases heart rates

Neurogenic inflammation—swelling on an autonomic basis

Reflex sympathetic dystrophy—neurogenic inflammation with severe pain

Migraine headaches—autonomically mediated abnormal dilation of brain blood vessels

Numbness, tingling, burning—when abnormal vascular tone or neurogenic inflammation presses on nerves or activates their sensors

Livedo reticularis and palmar erythema—loss of autonomic control in capillaries under the skin and increased flow through small, superficial arteries

---

patients becoming acutely aware of normal bodily activities. Patients report being uncomfortable as they feel palpitations or experience spasm in the abdomen, or have difficulty tolerating daily noises.

SUMMING UP

Regulation of autonomic control may be abnormal in fibromyalgia. Autonomic dysregulation can mimic some features observed in autoimmune disease and is often mistaken for them. Many commonly observed complaints in fibromyalgia, such as irritable colon, mitral valve prolapse, and tension headaches, are due in part to abnormalities of the ANS.

Part III

HOW AND WHERE THE BODY CAN BE AFFECTED BY FIBROMYALGIA

*I have been a frozen wretch my whole life, hardly able to
stand a whiff of wind or pain. . . . My rheumatic pains leave
me no rest. . . . I suffer stomach aches most of the time. . . .
My headaches are so terrible that life seems filled with
bile . . . paralyzing fatigue. . . . It is possible that I am more
seriously ill than my doctors think. The pain will not go away.*
Letters of Alfred Bernhard Nobel (1833–1896)

Fibromyalgia is known for its diversity of symptoms and signs. Every part of the body can be involved, and many of these manifestations are frequently misunderstood. This part discusses the more important symptoms and signs reported by fibromyalgia patients. Most of these complaints are complemented by case studies that illustrate the contexts in which they are most commonly encountered.

8

Generalized Complaints

Complaint is the largest tribute Heaven receives.
Jonathan Swift (1667–1745),
Thoughts on Various Subjects, 1711

Fibromyalgia is a syndrome rather than a disease, and as such has a variety of features. Any part of the body can be involved, especially when fibromyalgia is induced or aggravated by multiple factors. This chapter will review some of the generalized complaints expressed by fibromyalgia patients and place them in perspective.

CONSTITUTIONAL SYMPTOMS AND SIGNS

One of the major problems fibromyalgia sufferers encounter is difficulty communicating how they really feel. Complaints can be subjective and hard to verify or quantify. They consist of *symptoms*, or expressions of what is bothersome, and *signs*. Physical signs are observed during a physical examination, such as a rash or an irregular heartbeat, and are easier to validate. Constitutional symptoms or signs are generalized and do not belong to any specific organ system or region of the body.

Fatigue

Jane was an anthropology graduate student. In addition to carrying a full load of classes, she moonlighted as a waitress 20 hours a week. This pace was maintained until Jane caught what seemed to be a bad case of flu with a sore throat, runny nose, cough, fever, aching, fatigue, and swollen glands. Although most of her flu symptoms disappeared after several weeks, Jane never felt the same. The fatigue and aching became more pronounced, and Jane had to quit her waitressing job. She forced herself to go to class and was so exhausted that she spent most weekends in bed. Despite all of the bed rest, Jane never slept well and began noticing stiffness and spasm in her upper back and neck areas. The Student Health Service referred her to an internist, who ordered tests, all of which were normal. Jane now paces herself with rest periods alternating with active ones, avoids daytime sleeping, takes cyclobenzaprine (Flexeril) 2 hours before retiring at night, and engages in a general conditioning program. Even though Jane still is unable to work, at least she did not have to drop out of school. Fatigue is still a major problem, but its level of intensity seems to be slowly diminishing.

As with Jane, generalized fatigue is a prominent feature of fibromyalgia. Between 60 and 80 percent of fibromyalgia patients complain of *fatigue*, which is defined as physical or mental exhaustion or weariness. However, there are many reasons for fatigue. In a recent survey, 20 percent of the women in the United States and 14 percent of the men rated themselves as being significantly fatigued. This feeling can come on like a wave or be continuous.

Some of the basic causes of fatigue include emotional stress, depression, physical illness, poor sleeping, and poor eating. Examples of fatigue-inducing conditions include working too hard, substance abuse, anemia, low thyroid level, side effects of medication, overtraining, menopause, pregnancy, diabetes, heart disease, kidney impairment, cancer, depression, excessive perfectionist tendencies, autoimmune disease, and inflammation.

The majority of patients with fibromyalgia and chronic, otherwise unexplained fatigue in whom a primary psychiatric diagnosis has been ruled out also meet the criteria for chronic fatigue syndrome (see Chapter 13).

Do fibromyalgia patients run fevers?

Amber was having difficulty explaining what she meant. Until she was diagnosed as having fibromyalgia, she told doctors about her fevers. She related that it felt as if she was burning up or breaking out into a cold sweat. Physicians would obtain a normal temperature, look for infection, and inform her that they could not find anything. Although she never took her temperature during these episodes, Amber recalled her mother explaining that 97.4°F was normal for her and that when she had a temperature of 98.4°F it was a fever. Nobody believed her until a rheumatologist explained that altered ANS activity in fibromyalgia produces a feverish sensation. However, if her temperature was higher than 99.6°F on an ongoing basis, something other than fibromyalgia needed to be considered.

Everybody has a temperature, but few people run persistent fevers. A *fever* is defined as a body temperature above 99.6°F. Occasionally, patients complain to their doctor about recurrent fevers and relate that their baseline temperature is usually 96–97°F. Therefore, the normal temperature obtained at examination is a fever. Twenty percent of fibromyalgia patients include fevers in their list of complaints. Many, in fact, feel feverish. Hot and cold sweats or the sensation of "burning up" are not uncommon in fibromyalgia patients and reflect dysautonomia (see Chapter 7). Verifiable, chronic fever is *not* a feature of primary fibromyalgia but an indication that another condition is causing fibromyalgia-like complaints. Inflammatory conditions, infections, and tumors should be sought out.

Swollen or tender glands

The body's lymphatic system is a network of glands or lymph nodes that assist veins in clearing up water and debris and returning fluid from the arms, legs, and other areas of the body to the heart area. An infection such as a sore throat can lead to swollen lymph nodes in the neck area. Chronic poor circulation can produce edema from poor lymph drainage or varicose veins in the legs. Most lymph glands are enlarged when we have a local infection, an inflammation, or a malignancy.

Twenty percent of fibromyalgia patients complain of having swollen lymph nodes. Many who have a postinfectious fatigue syndrome start out with swollen glands, but the glands are no longer enlarged by the time a fibromyalgia specialist is consulted. Those who are thin also have relatively prominent lymph nodes, a condition not associated with any disease. As with a fever, if the doctor can feel the lymph nodes in a given area, this is not due to fibromyalgia but represents a circulation problem, allergic reaction, infection, inflammatory process, cancer, or simply bodily thinness.

The perception of tender lymph glands is common in fibromyalgia and reflects allodynia. The glands themselves are not enlarged or abnormal under the microscope.

9

"I'm Stiff and Achy"—
Musculoskeletal Complaints

*I don't deserve this award, but I have arthritis and I don't
deserve that either.*

Jack Benny (1894–1974)

Patients with each of the 150 distinct rheumatic disorders frequently have over-lapping muscle and joint complaints. Weakness, myalgias, arthralgias, spasm, lack of endurance, and stiffness are prominent features of fibromyalgia that may be difficult to differentiate from other conditions. The prominence of complaints in this area is what frequently brings patients to a musculoskeletal specialist such as a rheumatologist, as opposed to an infectious disease expert, general internist, or endocrinologist.

MUSCLE FINDINGS: WEAKNESS, MYALGIAS, LACK OF ENDURANCE, AND SPASM

Abigail was devastated after the unexpected death of her younger brother at age 30. Her physical and mental health had seemed tenuous, but she managed to pull herself together for the funeral and the visits of relatives from the Midwest. When it was over, Abigail's coping skills began to fray. First, she began experiencing left-sided upper back pain and thought it was from lifting Aunt Minnie's suitcase when taking her to the airport. Abigail saw the chiropractor she had consulted three or four times over a 5-year period for similar backaches. However, this time the pain did not go away and spread to the right side. Dr. Johnson's manipulations usually "snapped things back into place," but this time they made her worse. Abigail became very concerned when her fiancé tried to take her to Myrtle Beach for a relaxing weekend and found that she was in agony whenever he hugged her. Although she had been an aerobics instructor, Abigail found it very difficult to do her morning exercise routine and after several weeks gave up. Trying to exercise was extremely painful. Innocent movements such as washing her back in the shower caused her muscles to tighten up and go into spasm. Dr. Johnson referred her to a rheumatologist, who diagnosed fibromyalgia and instituted a medication, education, and rehabilitation program.

Over 80 percent of fibromyalgia patients have muscular symptoms or signs. Aching in the muscles, or *myalgias*, is common in the upper or lower back and neck area. Myalgias are usually present on both the right and left sides and present as a dull, throbbing discomfort. *Spasm*, defined as an involuntary muscular contraction, is less common than the sense of tightness in muscles that seems like spasm. Muscular aches tend to worsen after exercise and activity and as the day wears on. The discomfort is generally more severe in the late afternoons and feels "flu-like."

What is going on in the muscles? As discussed in Chapter 5, the muscles are weak only if deconditioning is present. Areas of taut bands may be felt as tender points. Some fibromyalgia patients who once engaged in vigorous exercise complain that they feel exhausted after a short workout and no longer have endurance. How does this happen? Postexertional pain occurs when arteries in the muscle constrict and not enough oxygen gets to these areas. Exercise requires increased oxygen to the muscles, and the lack of oxygen produces muscle pain. Fibromyalgia patients don't use oxygen optimally and prematurely deplete their energy reserves. This leads to deconditioning and produces a vicious cycle that promotes a fear of exercise.

Myalgias should be differentiated from inflammation of the muscles, which is known as *myositis*, and other conditions associated with aching muscles. Inflammatory processes such as polymyositis or systemic lupus can mimic fibromyalgia, as can a low thyroid blood level, myasthenia gravis, multiple sclerosis, infections, and anemia. Common prescription medications infrequently induce side effects affecting muscles, which leads to aching or weakness. Examples of this include certain cholesterol-lowering preparations (e.g., lovastatin [Mevacor], atorvastatin [Lipitor], pravastatin [Pravachol]) and the gout medicine colchicine. Inflammatory myositis, hypothyroidism, and the above-mentioned drugs can produce abnormally high blood levels of the muscle enzyme creatine phosphokinase (CPK) or abnormal electrical tracings in muscles on an electromyogram (EMG). Sometimes patients with primary muscle disorders have fibromyalgia-like complaints that can be diagnosed only with a muscle biopsy.

SOFT TISSUE AND JOINT COMPLAINTS: WIDESPREAD PAIN, ARTHRALGIAS, AND STIFFNESS

Janice was sure she had arthritis. Her mother could always tell when it was going to rain, and now Janice seemed to have this meteorologic prowess. As the day progressed, she would feel as if her body was stiffening up. Janice began noticing aching with pain in her shoulders and the back of her neck, particularly if she was premenstrual or had slept poorly. Janice felt much older than her 40 years. Her family doctor could not find any evidence of arthritis on examination or blood testing, and X-rays of her neck and shoulders were normal. Ibuprofen was prescribed, bringing temporary relief. Ultimately, it was concluded that Janice had a mild form of fibromyalgia that became evident when the weather changed, just before her period, and when she did not get enough sleep. Janice takes cyclobenzaprine (Flexeril) about three or four times a month when the discomfort starts to interfere with her ability to do things, but generally she feels well.

The International Association for the Study of Pain has defined *pain* as an unpleasant sensory and emotional experience. Widespread pain (from pain amplification) is such a prominent feature of fibromyalgia syndrome that it is included in the definition of the syndrome. The pain usually emanates from the soft tissues, muscles, and joints. Soft tissues include the supporting structures of joints such as tendons, bursae, and ligaments, as well as the myofascia. The myofascia lies between the lower skin (dermis) and muscles and consists of connective tissue and fat, which buffer muscles and provide structural integrity and support. The nature of the pain is highly variable. Some patients use descriptive terms such as *aching*, *burning*, *gnawing*, *smarting*, or *throbbing*. Pain can change sites and often gets better or worse on its own. Tender points are common in myofascial planes.

Fibromyalgia does not damage or inflame joints, but it can produce joint complaints. More than 80 percent of patients with fibromyalgia describe symptoms of aching in their joints, or *arthralgias*, and 60 percent have stiffness. Many patients also have other forms of arthritis, especially osteoarthritis, and a few have autoimmune disorders such as lupus or rheumatoid arthritis with a secondary fibromyalgia. A form of neck osteoarthritis, or being born with a narrow spinal canal, can lead to cervical spinal stenosis. This tightening of the spinal canal in the neck can be detected on an MRI scan and may aggravate the symptoms of fibromyalgia. Unlike degenerative osteoarthritis or rheumatoid arthritis, the arthralgias are not located primarily in the small joints of the hands or feet. In fibromyalgia, symptoms are usually prominent in the upper back, neck, shoulder, and hip areas. Other parts of the body, especially those that have been overused, can be involved. Whereas morning stiffness is an important feature of osteoarthritis and rheumatoid arthritis, most fibromyalgia patients become stiff in the late afternoon and early evening or when they have been in one position for a prolonged period of time. Stiffness is a difficult sensation to convey to others. Rheumatologists use the term *gelling* to denote the "jello"-like feeling of the stiff, tightened joints, muscles, and soft tissues of fibromyalgia. It improves when you move around, apply heat, or take a hot shower.

10

Tingles, Shocks, Wires, and Neurologic Complaints

The brain is a wonderful organ. It starts working the moment you get up in the morning, and does not stop until you get into the office.

Robert Frost (1874–1963)

Even though headaches, sleep disorders, cognitive impairment, burning, numbness, and tingling are potentially debilitating features of fibromyalgia, very few patients first consult a neurologist when they develop what turn out to be fibromyalgia symptoms. It has become apparent that the central, peripheral, and autonomic nervous systems play a more important role in fibromyalgia than was previously thought. This section will focus on these complaints and what causes them.

HEADACHE

Colleen had a splitting headache. Her temples were throbbing, and she could barely concentrate. When Dr. Smith prescribed Fiorinal, not only did the headache disappear but some discomfort in her upper and lower back that she had never bothered to complain about did also. Over the next few months, Colleen needed Fiorinal almost daily. Whenever she stopped taking it, the headaches returned with a vengeance. Dr. Smith referred her to a neurologist, who diagnosed Colleen as having fibromyalgia with associated "muscular contraction tension headaches." Colleen was told that the caffeine and barbiturate in Fiorinal helped her headaches in the short term but that continuous use resulted in "rebound" headaches from aspirin, caffeine, and barbiturate withdrawal. The neurologist stopped all her medication and helped Colleen "ride out" the withdrawal. She prescribed amitriptyline (Elavil) at bedtime for headache protection, and Colleen is now much improved.

Most fibromyalgia patients complain of recurrent headaches. These headaches usually are one of two types: tension or migraine.

Muscular contraction, or tension, headaches

Tension headaches are muscular contraction headaches. Patients describe these headaches as a dull "tight band around the head" similar to what they feel in other muscles of the body. Tension headaches and migraines are often associated with local elevations of substance P levels and decreased serotonin levels, stress, and low cellular pH (a more acidic cellular environment).

Tension headaches frequently involve the forehead, jaw, and temple areas. Occipital headaches, or pain in the upper part of the back of the neck, can be a type of tension headache and are associated with muscle spasm or stiffness. Osteoarthritis of the cervical spine can also cause occipital headaches. On occasion, moving the neck in any direction is painful. Tension headaches usually respond to the same remedies used to treat myalgias, arthralgias, and spasm.

Migraine headaches

Ten percent of the U.S. population suffer from vascular-mediated migraine headaches. Usually one-sided, associated with light sensitivity (photophobia), manifested by pounding, and preceded by a premonition of coming on, migraines occur in 20 percent of patients with fibromyalgia. Low serotonin levels are found in migraine sufferers, which in turn can alter vascular tone. Physiologically, a migraine begins with constriction of blood vessels (which produces the premonition, or aura) followed by dilatation. When arteries dilate, the stretching of the blood vessel and nerves evokes an intense headache.

Migraines are much more common in fibromyalgia patients who have ANS dysfunction. They complain of a throbbing or aching on one side of the head. This can be coupled with nausea or vomiting, visual disturbance (ocular migraine), or dizziness. Migraines can be brought on by unpleasant emotional stress, certain foods, menstruation, weather changes, smoke, hunger, or fatigue.

SLEEP ABNORMALITIES: NONRESTORATIVE SLEEP, SLEEP MYOCLONUS, BRUXISM

The alarm clock rang at 6 A.M., and Deidre felt as though she had never slept, even though she went to bed at 10 P.M. the evening before. She forced herself up and got ready for work. Deidre felt exhausted. This was happening with increasing frequency. Her initial response was anger—which she kept to herself. This seemed to tighten her head and neck muscles even more. That evening, Deidre decided to have two screwdrivers (vodka with orange juice) with dinner. She passed out at 9 P.M. and fell into a deep sleep. However, at 2 A.M. she awakened with palpitations and felt wired. Unable to get back to sleep, she made an appointment with her physician. Dr. Jones explained that nonrefreshing sleep is a common feature of fibromyalgia and that alcohol usually makes the problem worse, as does keeping anger to oneself. Deidre was given a prescription for nortriptyline (Pamelor) and joined the Arthritis Foundation, where she enrolled in their Fibromyalgia Self-Help course.

Sleep is necessary to promote the production of chemicals important in tissue growth and maintenance of immune function. As was mentioned in Chapter 6, nonrestorative (or nonrefreshing) sleep is found in most fibromyalgia patients. We all go through four stages of sleep, ranging from light to deep, where brain waves are denoted by the Greek letters alpha, beta, gamma, and delta. Persistent alpha wave intrusion into slow delta wave sleep results in waking up feeling sore all over and sometimes feeling more tired than when going to bed. Fibromyalgia patients make less growth hormone (which has little to do with growing in adults but is essential to maintain certain body functions) than healthy people while asleep, which can accelerate muscle injury and increase pain levels. These electrical abnormalities can be documented with a brain wave sleep study, known as a polysomnogram or a sleep electroencephalogram, which has been demonstrated in Figure 9.

Ten percent of patients with fibromyalgia also suffer from a poorly understood condition known as *sleep myoclonus*; their legs suddenly shoot out, lift, jerk, or go into spasm. Sometimes called *restless legs syndrome*, which also can occur when awake, this condition reflects a lack of oxygen in muscles and other tissues in the legs and is not unique to fibromyalgia. Additionally, some fibromyalgia patients grind their teeth when they sleep. Known as *bruxism*, this represents a tightening of the jaw muscles.

COGNITIVE IMPAIRMENT, OR "BRAIN FATIGUE"

Esther is a professional fundraiser whose mild fibromyalgia had been generally under good control. Friends and co-workers marveled at her ability to remember dates, phone numbers, and the names of everybody's spouses and children. Over the last few months, however, Esther had occasional difficulty recalling quickly some of the obscure facts that were her trademark. What amazed her was that nobody could tell the difference. Since her mother suffered from Alzheimer's disease, Esther consulted her mother's neurologist to make sure she did not have an early case. Her neurologic exam and an MRI scan of her brain were normal. Dr. Chapman ordered a single photon emission computed tomography (SPECT) scan, which suggested that some parts of the brain were not getting as much oxygen as they should. This reflected an abnormality in ANS regulation of blood vessel tone. Esther was told to pace herself during the day, with periods of activity alternating with four 20-minute rest periods, and was reassured. Dr. Chapman told her that if she did not improve, he could give her a low dose of fluoxetine (Prozac) and prescribe a cognitive therapy rehabilitation program.

Some of our fibromyalgia patients are concerned because they cannot think clearly, remember names and dates, balance their checkbook, or add numbers the way they once did. Characterized by confusion, memory blanks, word mix-ups, and concentration difficulties, these changes are often subtle and imperceptible to the physician who hears the complaint. Cognitive impairment, which some patients term "brain fatigue" or "fibrofog," is found in 20 percent of fibromyalgia patients. These complaints may be fleeting, intermittent, or constant and until recently were attributed to depression or stress. Additionally, some patients describe dizziness (which is not movement related), clumsiness and dropping things (which are not part of neurologic diseases such as multiple sclerosis), or visual changes or eye pain (which are not part of migraines). If these concerns are not handled wisely, patients are more likely to secondarily develop anxiety, panic, mood swings, and irritability.

Is cognitive dysfunction real, and how can we test for it?

For years, rheumatologists were as guilty as other doctors of ascribing cognitive impairment to depression or stress. How else could they explain the normal findings on neurologic examinations, MRI scans of the brain, and spinal fluid tests? However, on the basis of recent published work, we now know that cognitive impairment is real, and we are working hard to educate our colleagues.

Two lines of evidence provide support for the concept of nonpsychological cognitive dysfunction. First, in Chapter 6 we discussed the role of cytokines, chemicals that induce cognitive impairment along with fibromyalgia. Although our group and others have shown that cytokine blood levels are normal in this syndrome, evidence suggests that cytokine function is abnormally regulated. Second, by employing the SPECT imaging technique, Dr. Laurence Bradley and his colleagues at the University of Alabama have convincingly shown that fibromyalgia patients do not get enough oxygen to specific parts of their brain on an intermittent basis. Looking at the problem from a different angle, ANS abnormalities occasionally may produce enough spasm in cerebral blood vessels to deprive regions of the brain of oxygen. Interestingly, nonrestorative sleep by itself can produce these SPECT scanning abnormalities.

Serious, obvious cognitive dysfunction is uncommon, found in less than 5 percent of fibromyalgia patients.

NUMBNESS, BURNING, AND TINGLING

Frank managed a tire store that recently became computerized. He spent 2–3 hours a day "on-line" checking inventory and cash flow. When Frank began complaining of numbness and tingling in his hands, a co-worker suggested that it could be carpal tunnel syndrome. He consulted an ortho-

pedist, who gave him a wrist splint and injected the carpal tunnel region
with steroids. This was temporarily helpful. When Frank had his annual
physical with Dr. Grant, he told her about the numbness and tingling in his
hands but also mentioned that his feet felt numb at times as well. Dr.
Grant's examination revealed normal pulses and neurologic findings, but
some tenderness was elicited to palpation of the upper back, buttocks and
neck area. Dr. Grant ordered an EMG and a nerve conduction test, which
were normal. Since diabetes, a herniated disc, vascular disease, and carpal
tunnel syndrome were ruled out, Dr. Grant diagnosed Frank as having
myofascial pain syndrome with neuralgia. After 2 weeks of taking low-
dose amitriptyline (Elavil) and changing the position of his computer keyboard, the numbness was gone.

At some time, one-third of fibromyalgia patients will become aware of a vague
sensation of numbness, tingling, or burning. These symptoms may be reported in
any part of the body and tend to come and go. When neurologists are consulted,
their physical findings are usually within normal limits. Muscle and nerve blood
tests are also normal. Although diagnostic electrical evaluations with an EMG or
a nerve conduction study can identify cervical or lumbar disc problems, diabetes
or other metabolic abnormalities, inflammation, or compressive lesions such as
carpal tunnel syndrome, these studies are normal in primary fibromyalgia.
Carpal tunnel syndrome consists of compression of the median nerve at the
wrist as it enters the palm of the hand. Its prevalence is increased among fibromyalgia patients, especially those who work with computers all day and others
with poor workstation body mechanics. Carpal tunnel syndrome is usually
treated by splinting, local steroid injections, and, if needed, an occupational or
physical therapy evaluation. Anybody suspected of having carpal tunnel syndrome should have a confirmatory median sensory nerve conduction study of the
upper extremity before undergoing corrective surgery. Since hand numbness is a
feature of *both* fibromyalgia and carpal tunnel syndrome, some patients have had
expensive and unnecessary surgery that fails to relieve the numbness and tingling
of fibromyalgia. Unfortunately, we have observed the distinctive scar on the
inside surface of the wrist indicating carpal tunnel surgery in about 10 percent of
our patients, many of whom did not require surgery.

What causes painful nerve sensations in fibromyalgia?

Why should numbness and tingling be a feature of fibromyalgia? Painful nerve
sensations are a mild form of neurogenic inflammation or local nerve compression caused by autonomic dysfunction. Unless reflex sympathetic dystrophy is
present (see Chapter 13), it should evoke little concern. Although annoying and a
cause of aggravated poor sleep, fibromyalgia neuralgia (painful nerve symptoms)
never causes paralysis, strokes, or deformity. The management of numbness, tin-

gling, and burning is reviewed in Part VII, but the standard first-line therapy consists of tricyclic antidepressants such as amitriptyline (Elavil).

DRY EYES AND OTHER EYE OR EAR COMPLAINTS

Dry eyes or dry mouth, also known as *sicca symptoms*, have been reported in 10–35 percent of fibromyalgia patients. Manifested by burning, stinging, and redness of the eyes and verified by pits in the cornea on a Rose Bengal stain, diminished tearing in fibromyalgia has been attributed to altered autonomic nervous system activity. These small, difficult-to-see pits occur when the cornea does not receive enough moisture. Dry eyes are much more common than dry mouth.

Sicca related to fibromyalgia should be differentiated from an autoimmune-mediated dry eyes, dry mouth, and arthritis condition known as *Sjogren's syndrome*, in which autoantibodies are usually present. In Sjogren's syndrome, viral infections (as in AIDS or the mumps), alcoholism, and metabolic illnesses, the parotid (salivary) gland within the cheeks may become enlarged. Since tricyclic antidepressants are one of the principal treatments for fibromyalgia, and frequently cause dry eyes and dry mouth, it is sometimes difficult to ascertain how many people truly have fibromyalgia syndrome-induced dryness syndrome.

WHY AM I DIZZY? WHY DO NORMAL NOISES BOTHER ME?

More patients with fibromyalgia complain of feeling dizzy than otherwise healthy people. Dizziness can be a result of a bone spur in the neck causing pressure on the blood supply of the brain, chronic allergies with sinus inflammation, migraine, palpitations from autonomically mediated mitral valve prolapse, or a thyroid imbalance. Some fibromyalgia patients without these problems also notice a sensation of dizziness. Studies have suggested that the vestibular, or equilibrium, center in the ears is not optimally regulated in fibromyalgia patients. The reason is not well understood, but it may have to do with autonomic lack of blood flow to the vestibular center. Some fibromyalgia patients may have a low-frequency nerve-mediated hearing loss that is asymptomatic. Recent evidence suggests that these fibromyalgia patients are not really dizzy. Dizziness is a sensation of being in motion, but what some fibromyalgia patients are experiencing is *vertigo*, a malfunction of the vestibular center of the ear producing a sensation that everything around you is in motion. Some fibromyalgia patients have decreased noise tolerance on the basis of a hypervigilant vestibular reaction. Additionally, some fibromyalgia therapies, such as nonsteroidal anti-inflammatory drugs (NSAIDs), can lead to complaints of ringing in the ears, or *tinnitus*, or rarely, in other patients, diminished hearing.

11

Insights into Insides — Chest, Cardiovascular, and Other Concerns

The human heart is like a ship on a stormy sea driven about
by winds blowing from all four corners of heaven.

Martin Luther (1483–1546),
Preface to Psalms, 1534

Although some patients are concerned that their critical organs are involved in fibromyalgia, chest area symptoms infrequently are related to heart or lung disease. Palpitations, noncardiac chest pain, and subjective swelling or edema are important symptoms and signs of fibromyalgia. Reflux from the esophagus, gastrointestinal complaints, and female organ-related problems are also reviewed in this chapter in the context of fibromyalgia-associated concerns.

PALPITATIONS

The pounding in her chest was becoming unbearable, and Georgia was sure she would pass out. The sensation had been noticed before, but it usually stopped after several seconds. After several minutes, Georgia no longer felt lightheaded or dizzy. She broke into a cold sweat and heaved a sigh of relief. Her internist was aware of Georgia's intermittent musculoskeletal aches and spasms and fatigue, which were managed with ibuprofen and occasional cyclobenzaprine (Flexeril) at night. When Georgia mentioned her fatigue to Dr. Baker, her comments were greeted with silence and not immediately pursued. Consequently, she drank four Diet Cokes to make it through the work day in addition to her morning coffee. Dr. Baker ordered a two-dimensional echocardiogram (a heart imaging ultrasound) that demonstrated evidence of mitral valve prolapse. He told Georgia that the palpitations were brought on by drinking too much caffeine, and said that if she could not reduce her caffeine intake substantially, he would have to prescribe a beta blocker to control her heart rate.

The sense of having extra heartbeats, or *palpitations,* is reported in 10–20 percent of patients with fibromyalgia. Although heart disease, caffeine intake, anxiety, and other factors are associated with palpitations, many otherwise healthy young women have *mitral valve prolapse*. The prevalence of mitral valve prolapse is clearly increased in fibromyalgia. The mitral valve, one of the four valves of the heart that lies between its right-sided chambers, can become more floppy under ANS influence and produce palpitations. Patients feel as though they will pass out but rarely do. Mitral valve prolapse is also associated with chest pains and shortness of breath and can be easily diagnosed by an heart ultrasound known as a *two-dimensional echocardiogram*. Most patients with mitral valve prolapse do not require medication, and benefit from avoiding caffeine and learning how to relax. However, between 5–10 percent of these patients are referred to a cardiologist because they have potentially serious heart irregularities and may benefit from the initiation of heart drugs known as *beta blockers*.

COSTOCHONDRITIS AND NONCARDIAC CHEST PAIN

Hannah's father died from a heart attack when he was 50 and her favorite aunt at 46. Her serum cholesterol was a bit high, and she was 20 pounds overweight. Soon after Hannah celebrated her 45th birthday and was promoted to a high-pressure but prestigious position as head of sales for a cosmetics firm, it happened. Hannah developed chest pains and neck spasms so severe that she was sure the end was near. Her family rushed her to a community hospital. Hannah's electrocardiogram, chest X-ray, blood count, and chemistry panel were normal. However, her pain did not go away with nitroglycerine or Mylanta. When the doctor touched Hannah's third left rib at its juncture with the sternum (breast bone), she saw stars. Diagnosed as having costochondritis along with stress-induced fibromyalgia, Hannah was referred to an internist/rheumatologist for ongoing care.

As in Hannah's case, there is no question that costochondritis can be scary. The sternum, or breast bone, is connected to ribs by a rope-like tethering tissue. When this tissue (known as the *costochondral margin*) becomes irritated, it causes discomfort, especially in smokers, persons with lung disease or large breasts, and persons with inflammatory disorders such as rheumatoid arthritis. As noted in Figures 3 and 12, the costochondral margins are two of the tender points found in fibromyalgia. Sometimes referred to as *Tietze's syndrome*, this irritation produces chest pains. It sometimes takes an emergency room visit by a patient who is concerned about possibly having a heart attack before fibromyalgia is ultimately diagnosed. Costochondritis can be differentiated from cardiac pain because even though the sternum-rib attachments are tender to the touch, palpating the center of the sternum does not produce pain. A doctor may order chest or rib X-rays to make sure that there is no fracture.

Sometimes, patients with fibromyalgia report that it hurts when they take a deep breath. They fear it might be *pleurisy*, or irritation of the lining of the lung, which is extremely common in autoimmune diseases. Hannah did not have

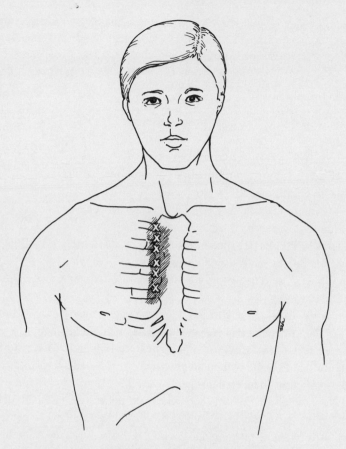

Fig. 12 *Costochondritis. The Xs mark potentially painful areas where ribs attach to the sternum.*

pleurisy, but this complaint reflects abnormalities in respiratory muscles that connect the ribs or irritation of the intercostal nerves located in that area.

Another form of noncardiac chest pain relates to the *esophagus* and is discussed in Chapter 13.

DOCTOR, CAN'T YOU SEE HOW SWOLLEN I AM?

Iris had been diagnosed with fibromyalgia. Premenstrually, her muscle and joint aches worsened and she gained 3–5 pounds. Over a 3-year period, Iris complained to several doctors that she felt swollen all the time. However, none of them found evidence of edema using the methods taught in medical school. One doctor bluntly and coldly told her that she was not swollen. A sympathetic internist prescribed Dyazide, a mild diuretic. Iris's fluid retention immediately lessened, but whenever she failed to take the medication, after several days her edema rebounded and became worse than ever. While on Dyazide, her muscle aching and spasms worsened. Her rheumatologist prescribed doxepin (Sinequan) for Iris's musculoskeletal aches, which resulted in an additional 10-pound weight gain. Ultimately, Iris was weaned off both medications.

One area of conflict we have observed between doctors and fibromyalgia patients involves the physician's skepticism that a fluid retention problem is really present. Women with fibromyalgia frequently report fluid retention and swelling. However, physical examinations and routine testing usually fail to document objective swelling. When doctors respond instinctively and prescribe a diuretic, or water pill, the fibromyalgia worsens because these preparations mobilize fluid by promoting muscle actions that induce more pain. Too many of these patients unfortunately become dependent on diuretics and gain 5–10 pounds within days when a different doctor or the patient stops the drug. Tricyclics in higher doses, particularly doxepin (Sinequan), can cause fluid retention as well.

Recent work from Great Britain has suggested that there is subclinical swelling, or fluid retention that is not noticeable on classic palpation, an electrocardiogram, chest X-ray, or pitting on physical examination. These studies provide evidence that in fibromyalgia autonomically mediated sympathetic nervous system hypofunction induces neurogenic vasodilatation (see Chapter 7). This leads to decreased arterial vessel tone, which produces decreased capillary flow and results in increased capillary leakage of sodium and water. The net result is a perceived loss of volume by the kidney, which reflexively secretes chemicals that promote salt and water retention, or edema. Premenstrual acceleration of this phenomenon is common.

SKIN COMPLAINTS

Some fibromyalgia patients have more than tender points under their skin. The skin itself is tender to touch. A manifestation of widespread allodynia, or heightened pain perception, this discomfort is present in more severe cases and is especially prevalent in patients taking steroids and in those who develop reflex sympathetic dystrophy (see Chapter 13).

There is no rash, per se, that is a unique feature of fibromyalgia. More patients than would be expected in the general population report dry skin, hair loss, itching, mouth sores, and easy bruisibility, although none of these complaints has yet been studied scientifically to determine if specific dermatologic problems are associated with fibromyalgia. Fibromyalgia patients also take more aspirin, ibuprofen, and other NSAIDs, which can result in black-and-blue marks under the skin.

As discussed earlier, autonomic dysfunction produces changes under the skin that mimic Raynaud's phenomenon and cause *livedo reticularis*, a lace-like mottling of the skin that usually produces no symptoms (see Chapter 7). It's not uncommon for fibromyalgia patients to have a ruddy complexion or red palms along with this condition.

GENITOURINARY COMPLAINTS

A variety of fibromyalgia-related conditions to be reviewed in Chapter 13 are associated with symptoms such as aggravation of premenstrual pain, the sensation of needing to void all the time, painful intercourse, and vulvar tightness.

GASTROINTESTINAL COMPLAINTS

Significant problems relating to the gastrointestinal tract, present in one-third of fibromyalgia patients, are part of the *functional bowel spectrum*, which is dis-

Table 5. *Prevalence (%) of Frequently Observed Symptoms and Signs in Fibromyalgia*

Widespread pain with tender points	100
Generalized weakness, muscle and joint aches	80
Unrefreshing sleep	80
Fatigue	70
Stiffness	60
Tension headache	53
Painful periods	40
Irritable colon, functional bowel disease	40
Subjective numbness, swelling, tingling	35
Skin redness, lace-like red skin mottling	30
Complaints of fever	20
Complaints of swollen glands	20
Complaints of dry eyes	20
Subjective significant cognitive dysfunction	20
Significant psychopathology	5–20
Nocturnal myoclonus, restless legs syndrome	15
Female urethral syndrome, irritable bladder	12
Vulvodynia or vaginismus	10
Concomitant reflex sympathetic dystrophy	5

cussed in detail in Chapter 13. Some of the major symptoms noted in this group of patients include diarrhea alternating with constipation, flatulence, distention, bloating, heartburn, stools with mucous, and diffuse abdominal pain.

SUMMING UP

A surprisingly wide range of multisystemic symptoms and signs in healthy-appearing people can be a source of frustration and misunderstanding among patients, family members, and physicians. Many of these complaints are part of regional fibromyalgia syndromes, or *fibromyalgia-associated conditions,* which are reviewed in the next three chapters. Table 5 lists the frequency of the principal complaints among fibromyalgia patients.

Part IV

THE CLINICAL SPECTRUM OF FIBROMYALGIA

Those who manage fibromyalgia respect its diversity of symptoms and signs. They appreciate and respect that it overlaps with other syndromes and disorders. Some of these conditions are, in truth, fibromyalgia masquerading under another name, and the very existence of others has been questioned. Local or regional forms of fibromyalgia add to the syndrome's complexity. This part will detail the manifestations that patients with these symptoms and signs experience and place them in the overall context of fibromyalgia syndrome.

12

*What Are the
Regional and Localized Forms
of Fibromyalgia?*

*Physicians think they do a lot for a patient when they give his
disease a name.*

Immanuel Kant (1724–1804)

The definition of fibromyalgia includes widespread pain in all four quadrants
(areas) of the body. What happens when you have fibromyalgia-like pain located
in only one or two quadrants of the body? Limited forms of the syndrome have
distinct features and terms used to describe them. *Myofascial pain syndrome*
encompasses many regional pain conditions ranging from temporomandibular
joint dysfunction in the jaw to a low back pain syndrome. The diagnosis of
myofascial pain syndrome requires that at least one trigger point be present and
that, when it is pressed, pain is referred to another site. This chapter will review
regional myofascial pain, relate it to fibromyalgia pain pathways, and discuss its
management and prognosis.

A BIT OF HISTORY: THE CONTRIBUTIONS OF
PHYSICAL MEDICINE SPECIALISTS

Our current concepts of tender points, trigger points, and regional pain amplification were developed by two of the best-known physical medicine thinkers,
Janet Travell and David Simons. Beginning in the early 1940s, Dr. Travell
became well known as John F. Kennedy's physician, who nursed him back to
health in the 1950s when back pain restricted his ability to walk. Later, she
became Lyndon Johnson's White House physician. Travell and Simon's textbook
on myofascial pain remains a classic and was updated as recently as 1992. Dr.
Travell (who died in 1997 at the age of 95) and Dr. Simons formed close working
relationships with rheumatologists, and their influence permeates every fibromyalgia study relating to tender points and regional pain.

Neurologists, neurosurgeons, and orthopedists diagnosed and treated localized muscle and nerve pain long before there were rheumatologists. At about the

same time that rheumatologists were becoming recognized and organized into a certifiable subspecialty, an equally small group of doctors were organizing themselves into a specialty known as *physical medicine and rehabilitation*. These doctors (who call themselves *physiatrists*) do not perform surgery, are not internists or family physicians, and do not manage autoimmune diseases. They concern themselves with areas not addressed by rheumatologists such as stroke, cardiac, and spinal cord injury rehabilitation. Physical medicine doctors usually practice in a hospital or hospital-like environment and work closely on a daily basis with physical therapists, occupational therapists, speech therapists, social workers, psychologists, and other allied health professionals. They supervise most of the inpatient rehabilitation centers in the United States. Although they have never numbered more than a few thousand, physiatrists have developed important insights into regional fibromyalgia-like pain that are reviewed in this chapter.

WHAT CAUSES REGIONAL MYOFASCIAL PAIN?

Most regional myofascial discomfort is produced by trauma. Unlike fibromyalgia, in which nearly 50 inciting factors have been implicated, localized or regional myofascial pain syndrome is usually due to either a single traumatic event or repetitive injury.

Numerous factors contribute to myofascial problems. The term *myofascia* refers to both muscles (myo-) and the *fascia*, the thin layer of tissue covering, supporting, and separating muscles. Abnormal posture can produce local discomfort. For example, scoliosis may be associated with midback or scapular pain on one side. A patient who has had lower extremity orthopedic surgery and needs to walk with a cane or crutch for a few weeks and is not used to it may place abnormal stress on the back, hips, shoulder, or elbow, resulting in a temporary regional pain syndrome.

From a physiologic standpoint, most of the neurochemical pathways reviewed in Chapters 4–7 play a role in regional body syndromes. However, in regional myofascial pain, more emphasis is placed on sensitization of a primary nociceptor, a nerve that receives painful stimuli and transmits that information to the spinal cord. This results in secondary hyperalgesia (more pain than would normally be expected in an area), allodynia (an ordinarily painless stimulus that produces pain), and/or referred pain. Pain that occurs from stretching a muscle is due to reflex spasm secondary to altered peripheral nociception elsewhere. Prolonged shortening of a muscle increases pain, as does overuse in the form of a sustained muscle contraction.

Referred pain relates to discomfort in areas that are near but not in the injured region or the affected tender points. Referred pain is produced by altered central nociception and enlarged receptor fields. It can be very misleading. For instance, suppose that an area on the left side near your midcervical spine is extremely uncomfortable. The traumatic insult that led to this condition might be in the back of the shoulder, but pain is referred to this area near the spine. For therapists, focusing rehabilitation energies on areas of referred pain is not as rewarding as dealing with the primary, inciting biomechanical problem. Figures 13–15 illustrate examples of referred pain.

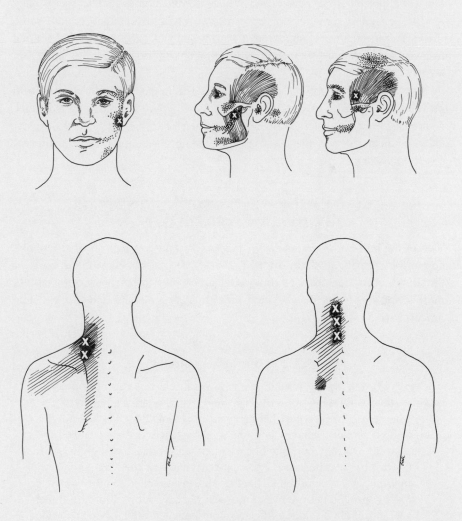

Fig. 13 (top) *TMJ dysfunction syndrome: tender points (X)*
and referred pain areas.
Fig. 14 (bottom left) *Upper back (trapezius) tender points (X)*
and areas of referred pain.
Fig. 15 (bottom right) *Occipital (back of the neck) tender points (X)*
and referred pain areas.

WHAT DOES A DOCTOR EXPECT TO SEE IN REGIONAL FORMS OF FIBROMYALGIA?

Patients with regional myofascial pain syndrome generally do not fulfill the ACR criteria for fibromyalgia. A distinct minority of patients with regional myofascial pain have systemic symptoms associated with fibromyalgia, such as fatigue, poor concentration, bloating, generalized weakness, and nonrestorative sleep. They tend to be slightly younger than most fibromyalgia patients and include more males. Pain occurs in an injured area long beyond its expected normal healing time and is chronic due to altered nociception or abnormal transmission of pain signals.

Myofascial pain syndrome can occur anywhere in the body, but more than 90 percent of these cases involve one of the following five regional combinations: neck and upper torso; temporomandibular joint (TMJ); neck, arm, hand; low back, buttock, leg; and the chest area, including costochondritis. See Figures 13–15 for examples.

EXAMPLES OF WELL-KNOWN SUBSETS OF REGIONAL MYOFASCIAL PAIN

Two of the best-known examples of regional myofascial pain involve jaw discomfort and repetitive strain disorder. Most TMJ patients consult ear, nose, or throat specialists, dentists, or orthopedists, as opposed to rheumatologists. In more serious cases, localized symptoms ultimately are connected to a systemic process such as fibromyalgia.

TMJ dysfunction syndrome

Dorothy began having trouble chewing meat, but this did not bother her since she was thinking of becoming a vegetarian. When she visited her sister's house and tried to play her niece's flute (something she had not done since high school), her left jaw felt as though it was being lanced by a sharp spear. Dorothy consulted her dentist, who found a very tight, tender TMJ. Dr. East sent her for a Panorex X-ray view of the TMJ, which was normal. She was diagnosed as having TMJ dysfunction syndrome. When Dorothy consulted her internist, Dr. Radford also noticed a lot of tightness and spasm on the left side of her neck and elicited a history of left-sided headaches in the back of her neck. Dorothy was started on ibuprofen, 600 mg three times a day, and was given jaw exercises and a muscle relaxant to take at night for a few weeks. A physical therapy referral was also given so that Dorothy could learn how to perform the exercises correctly, and a bite plate was fashioned for bedtime use. After 2–3 months, the TMJ symptoms eased. Dorothy now takes just ibuprofen occasionally.

Jaw pain is very uncomfortable and stems from many different sources. These include malocclusion, or an abnormal bite; arthritis of the joint (in rheumatoid arthritis and, to a less severe degree, in osteoarthritis); infection; bruxism, or teeth grinding; and traumatic injury. Myofascial pain from muscular spasm, with or without upper back and neck pain on the affected side, is a diagnosis of exclusion termed *temporomandibular joint dysfunction syndrome*. The pain stems from the same sources causing fibromyalgia and is amplified by anxiety, stress, or trauma, leading to unconscious jaw-closing movements. This regional form of fibromyalgia is diagnosed only after a dental evaluation and an ear, nose, and throat evaluation by a specialist, along with a special type of X-ray or imaging scan of the TMJ.

TMJ dysfunction syndrome afflicts 10 millions Americans; 70 percent are female. In a recent survey, 18 percent fulfilled the criteria for fibromyalgia and 75 percent of those with fibromyalgia had TMJ dysfunction. The temples, neck, and upper back can be affected. The TMJ dysfunction syndrome is treated with NSAIDs such as ibuprofen or naproxen, as well as moist heat, joint spacers (bite plates) worn at night, exercises, and a technique known as *spray and stretch* (see Chapter 19). Occasionally, injecting the TMJ joint with a small amount of steroid and a local anesthetic such as xylocaine may be useful. Most general management features that are reviewed in Part VI may also be recommended or prescribed. Once the diagnosis of TMJ syndrome is made, expensive and unnecessary surgery should be avoided except in extreme cases and only after several expert opinions are obtained.

Repetitive strain syndrome

Over the last few years, Geoffrey Littlejohn and his associates in Australia have performed pioneering work on musculoskeletal problems observed in the workplace. With Australia's generous worker's compensation system and excellent data collection methodologies, his group helped nurture our current concepts of repetitive stress syndromes. A discipline known as *ergonomics*, which is a hybrid of kinesiology (the science or study of movement), engineering, and physics, has explored the science of human performance at work. Practitioners have developed information about what types of local stress individuals can sustain in a work environment over a period of time. For example, working at a computer all day or lifting shipping cartons onto a truck are forms of repetitive strain, as illustrated in Jared's case in Chapter 3. Many patients in the former category might complain of pain in the shoulder, with numbness and tingling in the hand. Anti-inflammatory medication, physical therapy, and even a local injection of an anesthetic, with or without corticosteroids, is only temporarily beneficial if the fundamental ergonomics of the workstation are not adapted to the patient's requirements.

Some of these considerations, along with disability issues, are reviewed in more detail in Part VII.

If repetitive strain syndrome is not adequately addressed and the patient continues to engage in an ergonomically unsatisfactory job environment, not only might disability and chronic regional pain be the consequence but full-blown fibromyalgia can evolve.

WHAT'S THE PROGNOSIS?

The outcome of regional pain syndromes is generally very good to excellent, usually much better than that of fibromyalgia. Delays in treatment, incorrect treatment, or continued injury to the affected region have adverse consequences that can allow fibromyalgia to develop. The management of regional myofascial syndromes is outlined in Part VII.

13

What Disorders Are Associated with Fibromyalgia?

The fate of a nation has often depended upon the good or bad digestion of a prime minister.

Voltaire (1694–1778)

The perception of fibromyalgia as a distinct syndrome is relatively new. As recounted in Chapter 1, healers and sufferers have struggled to define what people have and how they feel with regard to widespread pain and fatigue complaints since the time of Job. Throughout this century, patients with fibromyalgia-like complaints have been diagnosed by physicians as having all types of conditions, syndromes, and diseases. Many of these overlap with fibromyalgia, and this chapter focuses on the most important ones.

CHRONIC FATIGUE SYNDROME

Friends always thought Kathy was an overachiever. They marveled that she could be an exemplary mother devoted to her two children and hold down a high-powered executive position while still finding time to run the church auxiliary and play tennis 6 hours a week. When she missed work for 3 days with a temperature of 102° F, a sore throat, cough, and swollen neck glands, nobody anticipated what followed. Although she returned to work the next week, it was clear that something had changed. Kathy was too tired to play tennis and started going to bed early. She began having difficulty thinking clearly and complained to her doctor about a "fog" in her brain. When the weather changed, Kathy reported being more stiff and achy. Ultimately, Kathy was diagnosed as having a postinfectious fatigue syndrome. She took a leave of absence from her job, but the company hired her as a consultant to help out with specific projects, which allowed her to work at a more leisurely pace. After 18 months, she returned to her job. Kathy seemed to be herself but was working at about 80 percent of her previous level.

The codification and "legitimization" of fibromyalgia with statistically validated criteria has paralleled similar initiatives concerning *chronic fatigue syndrome (CFS)*. Chapter 1 recounted some of the earlier insights and efforts.

An acute infection is often characterized by fever, swollen glands, and either a cold/bronchitis, a stomach/intestinal condition, or an aching/debilitating presentation. As the body fights infection and makes antibodies against microbes, acute symptoms and signs start to disappear and most of the time patients feel much better. However, a variety of organisms can stimulate the production of cytokines (discussed in Chapter 6) and other chemicals, which prolong fatigue and aching and may be associated with cognitive impairment, malaise, pain amplification, and sleeping difficulties.

How the Centers for Disease Control drew up criteria for CFS

Between 1930 and 1980, it was known that some patients recovering from infectious diseases such as polio, mononucleosis, and brucellosis had a prolonged convalescence and persistent systemic symptoms. By the early 1980s, a herpesvirus known as Epstein-Barr virus joined the group (mononucleosis is also a herpesvirus). For unknown reasons, it tended to afflict upwardly mobile young people, and the press tagged Epstein-Barr virus as a "yuppie flu disease." Epstein-Barr virus antibodies could easily be tested for, and its postviral fatigue complaints were treated symptomatically and waited out.

However, the "Epstein-Barr syndrome" epidemic turned out not to happen. The National Institutes of Health, United States Centers for Disease Control and Prevention (CDC), and other centers showed that over half of the U.S. population has evidence of exposure to Epstein-Barr virus in their blood, and standard antiviral therapy for herpes was not beneficial in these patients. Some Epstein-Barr patients had significant primary psychiatric problems, and numerous other organisms (e.g., bacteria, viruses, fungi, parasites) were shown to cause postinfectious fatigue syndromes. Chronic Epstein-Barr virus fatigue syndrome did exist, but it was overdiagnosed and in fact is relatively rare.

In 1984, I suggested in a medical journal article that fatigue syndromes and fibromyalgia could be one and the same. This hunch was documented when three world-renowned experts at Boston University tried an experiment. Drs. Anthony Komaroff and Dedra Buchwald, the most preeminent Epstein-Barr/chronic fatigue specialists in the United States at the time, had their clinic patients see a highly respected fibromyalgia expert, Dr. Donald Goldenberg. When Dr. Goldenberg's patients were sent to the Komaroff-Buchwald clinic, these doctors soon realized that the majority of their patients had both CFS and fibromyalgia.

The CDC devised statistically validated criteria for CFS in 1988, which were updated in 1994 (Table 6). The current definition of CFS requires unexplained, clinically evaluated fatigue of new or definite onset lasting for at least 6 months and not relieved with rest that substantially impairs performance. New onset of 4 of the following 8 factors must also be present: cognitive impairment, sore throat, tender cervical or axillary lymph nodes, muscle aches, joint aches, headache,

Table 6. *The CDC Revised Criteria for CFS (1994)*

1. Chronic fatigue of unknown cause that persists or returns for more than 6 months, resulting in a substantial reduction in occupational, educational, social, or personal activities.
2. The presence of 4 or more of the following symptoms concurrently for more than 6 months:
   a. Sore throat
   b. Tender cervical or axillary lymph glands
   c. Muscle pain
   d. Multijoint pain
   e. New headaches
   f. Unrefreshing sleep
   g. Postexertion malaise
   h. Cognitive dysfunction

sleep disorder, and malaise after exertion lasting longer than 1 day. By definition, patients with primary psychiatric disorders cannot have CFS. Using the aforementioned criteria, the prevalence of CFS in the United States is somewhere between 100,000 and 300,000, with several hundred thousand other persons having unexplained chronic fatigue without CFS. According to a study conducted in Great Britain, 4 percent of the population complained of chronic fatigue. If co-existing psychiatric and medical disorders were excluded, 0.5 percent of the population fulfilled criteria for CFS.

Sometimes, CFS is referred to as *chronic fatigue immune dysfunction syndrome (CFIDS)*. The authors prefer the term CFS since immune dysfunction is neither a proven nor prominent feature of the syndrome.

CFS and fibromyalgia: Similarities and differences

The majority of patients diagnosed with CFS in the United States are between the ages of 20 and 50, female, and Caucasian. Comparative surveys show that 20–70 percent of fibromyalgia patients have CFS, and 35–70 percent of those with CFS have fibromyalgia. CFS patients have greater elevations of antiviral antibodies than is observed in fibromyalgia. Whereas only a minority of fibromyalgia patients complain of a sore throat, show evidence of swollen glands or fevers, and have onset after a flu-like illness, these features are found in most CFS patients (Table 7). Although one well-regarded theory suggests that CFS is manifested after exposure to repeated viral infections in the setting of an overactive immune state, immune blood testing is inconsistent, contradictory, expensive, and does not change our treatment.

Autonomic dysfunction is common in CFS. This leads to low blood pressure in many of these patients, which is manifested clinically as *neurally mediated hypotension*, that aggravates fatigue. Cognitive impairment has also been docu-

Table 7. *Comparisons of fibromyalgia and CFS*

Parameter	Fibromyalgia (%)	Chronic fatigue syndrome (%)
Female sex	90	80
Muscle aches	99	80
Joint aches	99	75
Fatigue	90	99
Poor sleep	80	50
Complaints of fever	28	75
Complaints of swollen glands	33	80
Postexertional fatigue	80	80
Sudden or acute onset	55	70
Headaches	60	85
Cognitive dysfunction	20	65

mented with hypoperfusion on SPECT scanning, with the brain intermittently not getting enough oxygen.

THE FUNCTIONAL BOWEL SPECTRUM

Lilly always had a sensitive stomach, and whenever she was stressed it seemed that things ran right through her. As the vice president of a garment manufacturing company on the West Coast, she traveled to Asia at least once a month. Over time, Lilly developed frequent bouts of diarrhea alternating with constipation. She would be very gaseous, and her abdomen became intermittently distended. Lilly was sure she had picked up a parasite, and her internist, after obtaining normal blood and stool tests, referred her to a gastroenterologist. Dr. Sharp had also been aware of her complaints of mild aching and fatigue. He performed a colonoscopy and an endoscopy (procedures that allow a doctor to view the colon, esophagus, and stomach) and took biopsy specimens and cultures. Nothing was found. Lilly was started on hyoscyamine (Levsin), a drug that reduces intestinal muscle spasms and a higher-fiber diet, with substantial relief. She was diagnosed as having irritable bowel syndrome and returned to her primary care provider, who spent time with her working on lifestyle and dietary modifications.

The diagnosis a patient receives is usually influenced by the physician's background and training. For example, more than half of the internal medicine specialists in the United States have subspecialty training. Therefore, a patient who consults three different internists with training in infectious disease, rheumatology, or gastroenterology might be given a diagnosis of CFS, fibromyalgia, or functional bowel disease, respectively.

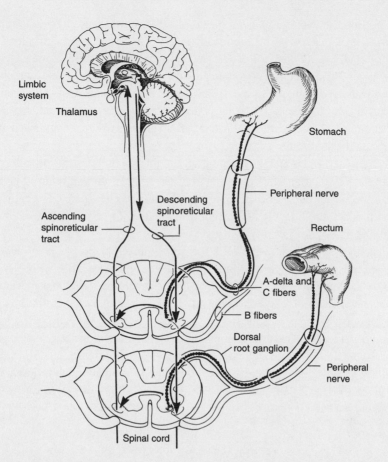

Fig. 16 *Visceral hyperalgesia. Functional bowel disease symptoms are thought to result from the amplification of parasympathetic nervous system B-fiber signals.*

Over the last decade, functional bowel disease has become a spectrum of gastroenterologic disorders with a common link of *visceral hyperalgesia*, or increased pain sensitivity in the internal structures. Identified by a variety of terms including *spastic colitis*, *irritable colon*, *diffuse abdominal pain*, *noncardiac chest pain*, and *nonulcer dyspepsia*, this spectrum was once primarily thought to be a motility, or movement, disorder. In fact, it has turned out to be a pain amplification disorder. Initiated by inciting factors that cause peripheral or visceral pain fibers and the parasympathetic nervous system to promote primary and secondary hyperalgesia with central sensitization, the functional bowel spectrum substantially overlaps with fibromyalgia. Recent evidence suggests that a neuropeptide found in the limbic system of the brain and the gut, cholecystokinin, produces abdominal or intestinal muscle spasms. Figure 16 illustrates these pathways.

Functional bowel complaints are the most common reason for referral to a gastroenterologist. As with fibromyalgia, 2 percent of the U.S. population fulfill the criteria for functional bowel disease, but as many as 20 percent may have it at some point. Patients report abdominal distention, bloating, pain relief with bowel movements, more frequent and loose stools with the onset of pain, frequent mucus in bowel movements, a sensation of incomplete evacuation, flatulence, and cramping. Some doctors believe that food allergies or medication sensitivity aggravate the syndrome.

Fibromyalgia complaints extend beyond the small intestine or colon. For example, sensitization of different parts of the spinal cord and referred pain can lead to persistent upper abdominal nonulcer pain and chest pains. Recent studies suggest that approximately 40 percent of patients with functional bowel disease fulfill the criteria for fibromyalgia and vice versa.

Functional bowel disease affects a type of muscle known as *involuntary*, or *smooth,* muscle. By contrast, fibromyalgia tender points overlie voluntary, striated, or skeletal muscle. Consequently, the treatment of functional bowel complaints involves dietary considerations (lactose restriction and more bulk), agents that diminish smooth muscle spasm (e.g., hyoscyamine [Levsin], dicyclomine [Bentyl], a hyoscyamine-atropine-phenobarbital combination [Donnatal]), preparations which promote bowel motility or decrease acid release (e.g., omeprazole [Prilosec], lansoprazole [Prevacid], cisapride [Propulsid]), and occasionally antibiotics or anti-inflammatory preparations. The role of diet in fibromyalgia is discussed in Chapter 18.

AUTOIMMUNE DISEASES

Ronna developed stiffness and aching in her hands and feet. At age 30, when Dr. Dale evaluated her, she looked great and the examination of her hands and feet was normal. Dr. Dale performed blood tests that showed slight anemia, a low white blood cell count, and a slightly elevated sedimentation rate (a blood test for inflammation). Dr. Dale told Ronna that her anemia was due to heavy periods and placed her on iron. Her low white blood cell count and elevated sedimentation rate could be explained by a cold she had 2 weeks before, and he told her to come back in 6 months. Ronna began developing pain in her upper back and neck area and started having muscle spasms. Six months later she had obvious swelling in her wrists and was markedly anemic; her white blood cell count very low and her sedimentation rate quite elevated. Dr. Dale did further testing that showed she had systemic lupus erythematosus, an autoimmune disease, on the basis of positive antinuclear antibody (ANA) and anti-DNA tests. He explained to her that her fibromyalgia-like complaints represented her body's reaction to the untreated inflammation of lupus.

Autoimmune rheumatic diseases are inflammatory processes in which the body makes antibodies to its own tissues, in essence becoming allergic to itself. On occasion, it may be difficult to differentiate these conditions from fibromyalgia. Untreated inflammation associated with autoimmunity may induce a secondary fibromyalgia, as might changing the doses of corticosteroids used to treat it. Surveys suggest that 7 percent of patients with Sjogren's syndrome, 15 percent of those with rheumatoid arthritis, and 22 percent of those with systemic lupus erythematosus have a secondary fibromyalgia.

Eosinophilic myalgia syndrome, eosinophilic fasciitis, and toxic oil syndrome

Maria worked as a flight attendant for an international carrier. To help her deal with jet lag, she frequently took L-tryptophan as a sleep aid during the 1980s. In November 1989 Maria developed a rash over her body and became short of breath. Her blood count showed high levels of eosinophils, a type of white cell, suggesting an allergic reaction. Antihistamines were of no benefit. Over the next few weeks, Maria's ankles swelled and the skin under her thigh started to become thick and felt like the outer surface of an orange. When her physician, Dr. Schiff, became aware of the publicity relating toxicity to L-tryptophan, she realized that Maria had eosinophilic myalgia syndrome. Upon taking prednisone (a steroid) for a few weeks, her symptoms and signs improved but new ones evolved. Numbness, tingling, and burning in her legs became symptomatic and within weeks were unbearable. Ultimately, her skin tightness, edema, breathing problems, and rash all disappeared or normalized. After a period of months, Maria developed multiple tender points and the chronic aching typical of fibromyalgia, along with widespread pain.

L-tryptophan is an amino acid that is converted into serotonin. In 1989, a contaminant in the manufacture of L-tryptophan (marketed as an over-the-counter sleep aid) produced a scleroderma-related autoimmune disorder known as *eosinophilic myalgia syndrome*. Several thousand people presented with high levels of eosinophils followed by muscle aching and abnormalities in the dermis and fascia, which produced swelling and tight skin. Most of these manifestations disappeared after patients stopped taking the drug, but after several months the majority of patients developed chronic fibromyalgia.

Over the years there have been rare reports of people who developed a syndrome identical to eosinophilic myalgia syndrome but never took L-tryptophan. Known as *eosinophilic fasciitis,* or *Shulman's disease* (named after Lawrence Shulman, a rheumatologist from Johns Hopkins), it is probably brought on by new, vigorous exercise routines in individuals whose serotonin is shunted in large amounts to the alternative pathway. One theory is that in some individuals, larger than normal amounts of serotonin are broken down by an alternative, or kynurenine, pathway, inducing anxiety and irritability. Other factors are also clearly at work.

Finally, an outbreak of eosinophilic myalgia syndrome-like disease occurred in Spain in 1981 after a manufacturer marketed adulterated, denatured rapeseed cooking oil. Follow-up studies of *toxic oil syndrome* among 15,000 people who became ill showed that many ultimately developed fibromyalgia.

LYME DISEASE

As a high school senior, Natalie was selected to attend a regional youth retreat in rural Connecticut. The mosquitos found her very attractive, and she noticed a quarter-sized, expanding red rash on her left leg a week after she returned to Manhattan. Nevertheless, she felt well and the spot faded. Several weeks later, Natalie developed flu-like symptoms and complained of muscle and joint aches. The results of the blood tests performed by her physician, Dr. Garth, strongly suggested Lyme disease, and he gave her antibiotics in high doses for several weeks. Except for some fluid in her right knee that had to be drained, Natalie seemed to improve overall, but she never felt quite the same. She noticed increased sensitivity to changes in the weather and on being touched, difficulty getting a good night's sleep, and increased anxiety. Dr. Garth diagnosed her condition as post-Lyme fibromyalgia. Natalie did not need additional antibiotics and was prescribed Sinequan drops at bedtime, which she took regularly for a few months and now uses only occasionally.

Since the mid-1970s, physicians have known that a deer-borne tick, *Ixodes dammini*, can infect people with a spirochete bacterium known as *Borrelia burgdorferi*. The disease was named for the area around Lyme, Connecticut, where it was first described; 90 percent of all cases are reported in the New England and mid-Atlantic regions.

Lyme disease is a complex malady. It presents in three stages. About one-third of tick bites are followed within a month by a distinct rash known as *erythema chronicum migrans*. Several weeks later, patients develop a generalized flu-like condition that may include joint swelling, muscle and joint aches, headache, sore throat, cough, fever, and swollen glands. If they are not treated with antibiotics (and infrequently if they have been treated), about 10 percent of the original group go on to a third stage in which potentially serious heart or nervous system involvement can develop.

What does fibromyalgia have to do with Lyme disease? First, a postinfectious fatigue/fibromyalgia syndrome ultimately afflicts a minority of Lyme disease patients. Second, many people who were told they had Lyme disease in fact had fibromyalgia. The reasoning is similar to what has been related about the Epstein-Barr virus. Blood tests for Lyme disease are not very reliable for diagnosing the disease, and many patients who consult a doctor for fibromyalgia-like symptoms have evidence of prior exposure to the Lyme disease–inducing spirochete bacterium. Does this simply represent being in an endemic area where many residents have been exposed, or is the condition actually a postinfectious Lyme fibromyalgia? There is an important reason to try to determine this. Patients who have evidence of Lyme disease should receive a course of antibiotics in order to prevent the more serious third stage of the disease. However, this expensive and time-consuming therapy is rarely necessary. Newer blood tests for Lyme disease are becoming available, which should help resolve this dilemma. If a primary care physician is not sure what to do, rheumatology or infectious disease specialty evaluations may be useful.

REFLEX SYMPATHETIC DYSTROPHY

It was a freak accident. Olivia was riding in a golf cart with her husband when he swerved to avoid a large rock and the cart overturned. She dislocated her left shoulder and underwent emergency surgery to repair it. Even though the repair was technically perfect, Dr. Bryan was concerned when her left hand swelled, the left shoulder remained immobile, and Olivia's excruciating pain persisted. A few days later, her right hand became swollen even though that side had not been injured. Dr. Bryan diagnosed her with reflex sympathetic dystrophy, injected her left shoulder with cortisone, and initiated a vigorous physical therapy program for her frozen shoulder. High doses of prednisone (a steroid) were also prescribed for 10 days. Despite this therapy, Olivia's shoulder had to be manipulated under anesthesia so that she could move it. Although the swelling improved over the following months, Olivia's burning, tingling, and generalized musculoskeletal discomfort were intense. Dr. Bryan referred her to a pain management center, which used several simultaneous modalities. Olivia's condition is slowly improving.

Reflex sympathetic dystrophy (RSD) can be induced by trauma, surgery, or certain drugs, or may occur spontaneously. A patient initially notices burning, tingling, and throbbing, sensitivity to touch or cold, and swelling of an arm or leg. A thorough examination usually demonstrates that both sides of the body are involved, although one side is more swollen than the other. The skin may be red or mottled. The affected extremity is painful to the touch and difficult to move. At first, a doctor may suspect a rheumatoid-like inflammatory arthritis. The swelling represents a form of neurogenic inflammation (see Chapter 7). In the second phase of RSD, the swelling becomes brawny and thicker, with pigment changes 3 to 6 months later. The numbness, burning, and tingling persist. After 1

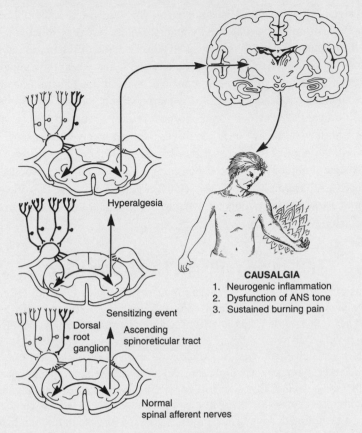

Hyperalgesia

Sensitizing event

Dorsal
root
ganglion

Ascending
spinoreticular tract

Normal
spinal afferent nerves

CAUSALGIA
1. Neurogenic inflammation
2. Dysfunction of ANS tone
3. Sustained burning pain

Fig. 17 *Reflex sympathetic dystrophy. Amplified musculoskeletal pain is complicated by ANS reactions that lead to severe burning, pain, and swelling.*

or 2 years, muscle atrophy and wasting are evident in the affected limb, affected bones become osteoporotic (termed *Sudeck's atrophy*), and range of motion may be decreased. The swelling disappears, but a chronic pain syndrome with generalized fibromyalgia develops. A milder, regional RSD known as *shoulder-hand syndrome* is associated with a frozen or immobile shoulder.

RSD is a form of sympathetically mediated pain. Officially designated as a "complex regional pain syndrome," it afflicts 1 person in 5000. Occurring when peripheral sensory receptors are oversensitized or outgoing sympathetic impulses are short-circuited to incoming sensory fibers, RSD can be a type of *causalgia*, consisting of sustained burning pain with allodynia, increased reaction to a stimulus, and dysfunction of autonomically mediated blood vessel tone. In RSD, chronic nociceptive stimulation produces sympathetic nervous system reactions (illustrated in Figure 17). This painful condition is very frustrating and difficult to treat. RSD probably represents 1–2 percent of fibromyalgia patients in a community rheumatology practice.

In its early phase, RSD should be managed aggressively with short courses of high-dose corticosteroids, vigorous mobilization, and physical therapy. Once RSD has entered the second stage, some of its chronic features are irreversible. Although the approaches used to treat fibromyalgia discussed in Part VI are useful, two additional aspects of RSD therapy need time and careful consideration. First, prolonged, aggressive physical therapy is helpful. Preferably, this should be prescribed in consultation with a physical medicine and rehabilitation specialist or orthopedist. Local steroid injections and sympathetic nervous system blockade are frequently helpful. Second, RSD patients may require narcotic pain medication in order to make it through the day, and a pain management consultation with follow-up may be advisable.

RSD patients are probably in more pain for longer periods of time than patients with most other rheumatic diseases. Once an RSD patient enters the second phase of the disease, a multidisciplinary approach is optimal: consultants from various specialties who communicate regularly to coordinate care provides the highest level of comfort and the best outcome for this unfortunate group of people.

PREMENSTRUAL SYNDROME AND DYSMENORRHEA

Naomi had a tendency to be stiff, achy, and tired. All of her blood tests were normal, and she was diagnosed as having fibromyalgia on the basis of her history and tender points on examination. Most of the time the condition was mild and required no treatment. However, the symptoms greatly worsened a few days before her period started. Naomi became very irritable and difficult to talk to. She once failed a final exam in history, even though her mastery of the material was obvious, because of inability to concentrate. Naomi was concerned that she could lose her after-school sales job due to the mood swings related to *premenstrual syndrome* (*PMS*) that disturbed her co-workers and customers. Dr. Tash successfully treated Naomi with a combination regimen of ibuprofen and diuretics taken for 3 days every month premenstrually along with a muscle relaxant in the evening.

The release of hormones, prostaglandins, and other chemicals along with seratonin dysfunction prior to the onset of menses can cause fluid retention, a sense of bloating, alterations in mood and behavior, and occasionally painful periods (dysmenorrhea). While most women experience these cyclical alterations, 3–10 percent of American women have severe physical and psychological symptoms that interfere with their ability to function. They complain of irritability, tension, headache, backache, breast tenderness, depression, lack of energy, difficulty concentrating, a sleep disorder, and feeling "out of control." About 70 percent of women with fibromyalgia experience flares premenstrually, and the prevalence of fibromyalgia among those with more severe dysmenorrhea is increased. In addition to managing fibromyalgia, treating doctors frequently add an ibuprofen- or naproxen-containing anti-inflammatory agent to be taken a few days just before the onset of menstruation. Other women report relief when they take a mild diuretic (water pill) for these few days as well.

FEMALE URETHRAL SYNDROME, OR IRRITABLE BLADDER

Almost every hour Sherrie had to urinate, regardless of attempts at control. Sherrie seemed to have many bladder infections that never responded fully to antibiotics, although she always felt better while being treated. She often felt an intense, sudden urge to void, even though only dribbling occurred. Finally, her family physician referred Sherrie to a urologist. Dr. Stern obtained negative urine cultures. An X-ray known as an intravenous pyelogram (IVP) failed to demonstrate structural abnormalities in the kidney, ureter, or bladder. Dr. Stern performed cystoscopy (examining the bladder through a telescope inserted into the urethra) and found no inflammation, polyps, or tumors. There were no strictures in the urethra. Sherrie visited her family doctor a few weeks later because of tension headaches and muscle aches. Dr. Jones thought these symptoms were from a myofascial source. He prescribed cyclobenzaprine (Flexeril) at night, which, incidentally, greatly diminished her urge to void. At her next visit to Dr. Stern, he informed Sherrie that she was suffering from female urethral syndrome and added oxybutynin (Detrol) to take during the day.

Among young women, urinary tract infections are extremely common. All too often, in order to make it convenient for the doctor and the patient, antibiotics are prescribed by telephone for symptoms and signs of burning with voiding, blood in the urine, or frequent urination. In an ideal world, antibiotics should be prescribed after a urine culture is obtained, and the prescription might be altered 48 to 72 hours later when the infecting organism has been grown and identified. Some patients have recurrent infections, and still others are on chronic antibiotic prophylactic therapy.

Within this population, a subgroup of young women fall through the cracks. They complain of intense pain with urination, and the urinalysis may show a few pus cells or red blood cells. The urine cultures are always negative, and mechanical problems such as a urethral stricture or neurogenic bladder are not present. Sometimes the pain seems to lessen with an antibiotic, although this is usually because doctors frequently add anesthetic medicines (e.g., phenazopyridine [Pyridium]) to the antibiotic, which diminishes discomfort while voiding. These patients have *female urethral syndrome*, which our group was the first to associate with fibromyalgia. Representing spasm of the muscles around the urethra, an irritable bladder is found in 10–15 percent of fibromyalgia patients. Its management consists of reassurance, avoiding antibiotics, phenazopyridine hydrochloride [Pyridium] (a urinary anesthetic), and antispasmodics (e.g., oxybutynin [Ditropan, Detrol]). We have found that when muscle relaxants such as diazepam (Valium) or cyclobenzaprine (Flexeril) are taken for a few nights, urethral spasm usually abates for periods ranging from days to months.

VULVODYNIA AND VAGINISMUS

Paulette was 11 when her stepfather molested her after drinking heavily. She was very frightened and did not tell anyone. As a young adult, her dating experiences were characterized by perfunctory, unenjoyed sex and difficulty forming close relationships. With time, her vaginal muscles tightened so much that penetration was impossible, and her vulvar area always hurt. Paulette's gynecologist could not find any structural abnormalities, tumors, or infection. Paulette never discussed these complaints with her internist, who had already diagnosed her with fibromyalgia on the basis of headaches, difficulty sleeping, aching, and fatigue. When her stepfather developed terminal cirrhosis of the liver, Paulette's fears and anxiety increased. She met with her internist, told her the whole story, and was referred for counseling. As a consequence, Paulette finally told her mother and sister what had happened. Her vulvar pain and vaginal tightness decreased, as did her fibromyalgia. She finally confronted her stepfather. Even though he denied everything, Paulette was finally able to obtain closure and get on with her life.

Seen in less than 5 percent of fibromyalgia patients, intense discomfort in the female genital tract can reflect a painful vulva (the visible external female genital area) without infection or other pathology (*vulvodynia*) or involuntary spasms of the vaginal muscles when entry is attempted (*vaginismus*). This results in painful intercourse and has serious lifestyle implications. Many of these women also have female urethral syndrome. Studies have shown that many women with vulvodynia or vaginismus have a history of sexual or physical abuse, a rape experience, or psychological problems especially related to feelings of guilt, anger, fear, or loss of control. In our experience, pain amplification, or fibromyalgia, can be a complication of sexual or physical abuse, but this is *not* found more commonly in the 95 percent of fibromyalgia patients without vulvodynia or vaginismus (see Table 8). In addition to prescribing medication to manage fibromyalgia, we advise our vulvodynia or vaginismus patients to seek counseling with an understanding sex therapist and/or psychologist experienced in this sensitive area. A recent report has suggested that biofeedback to the pelvic floor musculature ameliorates some of the symptoms.

Table 8. *Fibromyalgia-associated conditions*

Condition	% who have fibromyalgia	% with fibromyalgia who have associated conditions
Chronic fatigue syndrome	50	50
Functional bowel	20	40
Autoimmune disease	10	2
Lyme disease	30	2
Reflex dystrophy	100	5
Premenstrual syndrome	10	50
Female urethral syndrome	10	12
Vulvodynia, vaginismus	50	5
Mitral valve prolapse	10	20
Tension headache	20	53
TMJ dysfunction	18	75
U.S. population	2	—

STEROID, HEROIN, ALCOHOL, OR COCAINE WITHDRAWAL

Ursula experienced a lot of aching in her hands and feet. At age 23, she was too young to develop arthritis. Dr. Abel could not find anything on examination and told Ursula to take Orudis KT (an over-the-counter aspirin-like anti-inflammatory drug) when she felt pain. One month later, her knuckles began to swell, and upper back and lower buttock pain developed. Dr. Abel diagnosed her with early rheumatoid arthritis on the basis of Ursula's examination and the presence of rheumatoid factor in her blood. He also found myofascial tender areas in her upper and lower back regions that he explained would disappear with treatment. He was absolutely correct. Ursula took methotrexate, and her rheumatoid arthritis and fibromyalgia pains went away. After 6 months, however, blood test abnormalities forced Dr. Abel to stop the methotrexate and substitute low doses of prednisone (a steroid). When Ursula's rheumatoid arthritis continued to be stable, he decreased the dose of prednisone from 10 to 5 mg a day. Four days later, Ursula's myofascial tender points became unbearable but her rheumatoid arthritis stayed quiet. Dr. Abel prescribed amitiyptyline (Elavil) for a few nights until her steroid-withdrawal fibromyalgia resolved.

Corticosteroids are prescribed for a variety of inflammatory and allergic conditions ranging from asthma, ulcerative colitis, and sinus irritation to rheumatoid arthritis and lupus, and along with chemotherapy for certain malignancies. When steroids are taken for more than a few weeks, the skin becomes very sensitive to touch or pressure. It also becomes sensitive to small alterations in steroid doses. For example, if a patient is taking 15 mg of prednisone and the dose is reduced to 10 mg, the decrease in dose can produce a *steroid withdrawal fibromyalgia*. This is not classical fibromyalgia because if the dose stays at 10 mg, most of the fibromyalgia-like pain and spasm disappear within a few weeks. Long-term steroid administration is associated with secondary fibromyalgia by causing increased skin and soft tissue sensitivity.

Acute, transient circumstances in which a temporary fibromyalgia-like situation occurs are also found in patients withdrawing from alcohol, heroin, or cocaine.

TENSION HEADACHE SYNDROME AND MITRAL VALVE PROLAPSE

Headaches are a common feature of fibromyalgia. Detailed histories indicate that many patients who seek neurologic consultation for tension headaches turn out to have fibromyalgia symptoms and signs. We discuss tension headaches in Chapter 10 and mitral valve prolapse in Chapter 11.

SUMMING UP

Pain amplification, widespread pain, and systemic symptoms are not unique to fibromyalgia; variants of these three symptoms are found in many other conditions. Some conditions overlap with fibromyalgia to varying degrees and are managed with similar treatment approaches. Table 8 summarizes some of the relationships between fibromyalgia-associated conditions.

14

Controversial Syndromes and Their Relationship to Fibromyalgia

It's no longer a question of staying healthy. It's a question of finding a sickness you like.

Jackie Mason (1931–)

Over the years, a variety of health professionals have developed terms or phrases to denote seemingly unique clinical combinations of symptoms and signs. A disorder or syndrome does not necessarily exist simply because it has been described in the medical literature. Some have stood the test of time, others overlap with syndromes described by different specialists, and additional terms may be favored by a single practitioner advocating a "cause." This chapter reviews conditions that have overlapping features with fibromyalgia but are not yet regarded as full-blown, legitimate disorders by organized medicine.

ALLERGIES AND "MULTIPLE CHEMICAL SENSITIVITY SYNDROME"

When Dr. Fine first met Wanda, she was a basket case. Wanda had canceled three prior appointments because smells from a new carpet had made her sick, Med fly agricultural spraying 30 miles away prevented her from getting out of bed, and she developed a severe headache when her neighbors' house was being painted. She almost passed out in the elevator going to Dr. Fine's office because somebody was smoking. Wanda had been to three allergists, who obtained normal skin tests and blood tests. Desperate, she traveled to Mexico, where "immune rejuvenating" injections were administered, and to Texas, where a clinical ecologist sequestered her in a pollution-free, environmentally safe quonset hut for a month. There she received daily colonics, antiyeast medication, and vitamin shots, to no avail. Dr. Fine elicited a history of aching, sleep disorder, a "leaky gut," muscle pains, fatigue, and a spastic colon. His physical examination and mental status examination revealed evidence of anxiety, obsessive-compulsive tendencies, and fibromyalgia tender points. Wanda was treated with fluoxetine (Prozac) for pain and obsessive behavior, buspirone (Buspar), for anxiety during the day, and trazodone (Desyrel), a tricyclic, to help her sleep at night. She was referred to a psychologist who worked to improve Wanda's socialization skills and encouraged her to go out rather than be a prisoner in her own home. Wanda is slowly improving but will need many months of therapy.

Self-reported environmental sensitivities are observed in 15 percent of Americans. From 3 percent to 7 percent of fibromyalgia patients report extreme sensitivity to environmental components, particularly cigarette smoke, noise, bright lights, cold temperatures, pollution, gas, paint, perfumes, solvent fumes, pesticides, auto exhaust, certain foods, and carpet smells. A study conducted by the National Institutes of Health documented that one-half to three-quarters of patients with chronic fatigue syndrome (CFS) complain of having many allergies and sensitivities.

Multiple chemical sensitivity syndrome is a controversial entity. Proponents of the syndrome explain that it is triggered by exposure to diverse chemicals at doses lower than those documented to cause adverse affects in humans. *Cacosmia* is the subjective sense of feeling ill from low levels of environmental chemical odors. Cognitive impairment complaints are common. Interestingly, conventional allergy skin tests are often normal.

About 5 percent of allergists call themselves *clinical ecologists* and attribute many of our nation's ills to environmental sensitivities. They use terms such as *chemically induced immune dysregulation, food allergies, leaky gut syndrome, allergic tension-fatigue syndrome, allergic toxemia, 20th-century disease, ecologic illness,* or *yeast syndrome* to explain these conditions. This group is not recognized by organized medicine and has developed testing methodologies that are not endorsed by mainstream practitioners. The National Research Council and the American Medical Association have issued position papers stating that there is not enough evidence to recognize multiple chemical sensitivity as a clinical syndrome. Many highly respected allergy/immunology specialists believe that multiple chemical sensitivity syndrome is overdiagnosed; others do not think it exists. This controversy is mentioned only to explain why some fibromyalgia patients may be given mixed signals and contradictory advice by various specialists.

Unfortunately, there is no consensus within the discipline of allergy and immunology about how to best define and categorize patients with environmental complaints who relate that allergies or chemicals cause widespread pain and fatigue. The American Academy of Allergy and Immunology, the American College of Physicians (to which most internists belong), and the American College of Occupational Medicine have issued position statements that the clinical ecology literature provides inadequate support for their beliefs and practices. In other words, double-blinded, prospective trials (in which patients did not know what they were being tested for or treated with and half of whom received no treatment) have not borne out clinical ecology theories.

Most patients labeled as having multiple chemical sensitivity syndrome have nociceptive amplification as a form of fibromyalgia or CFS, while others have a primary psychological disturbance, primarily a panic disorder, which may play a role in these complaints. Additionally, we have had patients whose symptoms and signs disappeared with antiallergy therapies. A group at the University of Arizona has postulated that mutiple chemical sensitivity is not immunologic but is a form of hypervigilance that results from the ability of the olfactory neurons and the limbic system to amplify responses to chemicals in concert with a dsyfunctioning ANS.

The most important issue in treating patients with environmental sensitivities and allergies is to make sure that they do not become so fearful of going outside and living normally that they become "environmental cripples."

A subset of patients with chemical sensitivity developed their condition, known as *sick building syndrome*, or *building-related illness*, after a defined exposure. Because their fibromyalgia-like conditions evolved after exposure to specific chemicals found in structures, this group of patients usually has a better prognosis than the overall multiple chemical sensitivity group in general.

Patients diagnosed with multiple chemical sensitivity syndrome should have their fibromyalgia managed symptomatically (see Parts VI and VII). They should work closely with their allergist/immunologist once a primary psychiatric disorder has been ruled out or treatment has been initiated (see Chapters 17 and 20).

GULF WAR SYNDROME

A total of 670,000 U.S. soldiers served in the 1991 Persian Gulf War. A combination of symptoms characterized by fatigue (61 percent), joint pain (51 percent), nasal sinus congestion (51 percent), diarrhea (44 percent), joint stiffness, irritable colon, myalgias, and cognitive impairment (all 41 percent) and headache (39 percent) was reported by 17,248 military personnel. When strict criteria were applied (symptoms starting 2–3 months after leaving the Persian Gulf with a duration of more than 6 months, other diseases having been ruled out), probably 3000 military personnel had what has been called *Gulf War syndrome*. Gulf War syndrome may have been induced by giving combatants an insect repellent known as DEET in combination with pyridostigmine, an agent that minimizes the toxicity of nerve gas. Together, these drugs prolong acetylcholine activity and can produce some of the symptoms reported by the soldiers (see Chapter 7). Other mechanisms for Gulf War syndrome have also been proposed. One well-documented report found that 25 percent of Gulf War syndrome patients fulfilled the ACR criteria for fibromyalgia.

SILICONOSIS

After graduating from high school, Tanya worked as a model. Although men found her quite attractive, her modeling roommates teased her about her small breasts. As Tanya was an only child from a broken home, these taunts did not help her self-image. On an impulse, she consulted a plastic surgeon who promised to make her a "complete woman." Tanya underwent breast augmentation with a silicone gel prosthesis. For 5 years the result looked great and she had few regrets, although she had some mild upper chest discomfort and the surgery had eliminated all nipple sensation. Then, over 1–2 years, symptoms of fatigue, burning, tingling, and aching started to evolve. Her eyes were so dry that she began using artificial tears. When press reports about silicone were published, Tanya went to a rheumatologist. Dr. Silbart obtained a positive antinuclear antibody (ANA) test and found evidence of fibromyalgia on physical examination. A plastic surgeon suspected a right-sided implant rupture that was confirmed on an MRI scan. After the implants were removed, Tanya's symptoms improved for about 6 months and her ANA level dropped by half. Her plastic surgeon and psychiatrist attributed her symptoms to Tanya's underlying psychological problems and felt strongly that the implant rupture was coincidental. Dr. Silbart believed that implants played an important role in her medical problems, but another rheumatologist referred by a law firm agreed with the psychiatrist and plastic surgeon. Her internist was not sure, told Tanya that a combination of factors was causing her complaints, and reassured her in a way that minimized her anxieties and fears.

This controversial condition is based on the premise that the silicone in breast implants can be broken down to silica or related products, which spread throughout the body. For over 50 years, silica has been known to stimulate the immune system. Among exposed gold and uranium miners, silica occasionally results in the formation of autoantibodies and a scleroderma- or lupus-like disorder 10–30 years after exposure. *Siliconosis*, a term coined by Dr. Gary Solomon at New York University in the early 1990s, could be its cousin seen in some patients with breast implants. Many siliconosis patients have a fibromyalgia-like condition with chronic fatigue, muscle and joint pain, swollen lymph glands, dry eyes, cognitive dysfunction, and difficulty swallowing, with or without the presence of autoantibodies. Other physicians have countered that silicone is not broken down to silica, and they believe that the role of these symptoms and illnesses is no different in women without implants. In the current litigious atmosphere, it will probably be several years before these claims are sorted out in a scientifically acceptable fashion.

LEAKY GUT SYNDROMES

Irritable bowel, spastic colitis, and functional bowel disease are recognized disorders of visceral hyperalgesia (increased pain sensitivity in internal structures), along with altered gut motility, and were reviewed in Chapter 13. Over the years, some homeopaths, naturopaths, and other alternative medicine practitioners have hypothesized that when too many substances pass through the lining of the small intestine, it becomes more permeable than usual. In other words, an overload of toxins or poisons is present that overwhelms the ability of the liver to detoxify them. As a consequence, inflammation and infections, as well as hormonal and neuromuscular changes, ensue.

Known as the *leaky gut syndrome*, this disorder has been held to cause *reactive hypoglycemia,* or low blood sugar, which in turn can induce palpitations, low blood pressure, and a feeling of faintness. Only one study supporting this claim has ever been published in a quality medical journal (*The Lancet*), and it has not been confirmed. Leaky gut syndrome has been claimed to be aggravated by aspirin- and ibuprofen-like products, food allergies, and yeast. Standard medical textbooks do not mention the existence of leaky gut syndrome, and most mainstream physicians believe that the majority of these patients have functional bowel or psychiatric disorders.

Candida hypersensitivity syndrome:
A yeast connection or disconnection?

Candida hypersensitivity syndrome is a variant of the leaky gut syndrome, according to Dr. William Crook, a Tennessee family practitioner, who popularized the theories of Dr. C. Orian Truss in a 1983 best-seller, *The Yeast Connection: A Medical Breakthrough.* Yeast is a fungus known by the technical term *candida.* Verifiable yeast infections are present in healthy people, as well as being a complication of diabetes; pregnancy; progesterone, steroid, chemotherapy or antibiotic therapy; and altered immune states. Dr. Crook hypothesized that certain people develop hypersensitivity to a toxin released by yeast that exists naturally in the gastrointestinal tract, vagina, and respiratory tract. This, along with a lack of "good" bacteria, leads to a general feeling of ill health and to the same inflammatory, immune, hormonal, and neuromuscular changes attributed to leaky gut syndrome. Dr. Crook advocated a diet with carefully controlled sugar, wheat product, and yeast intake, attention to food allergies, nutritional supplements, and anti-yeast medication.

Unfortunately, no controlled trials in the peer review literature support his claim, and when anti-yeast medication was given in a double-blind fashion (where half of the patients unknowingly took a placebo), no differences were noted. Yeast antibody tests are available in many clinical laboratories but consistently fail to identify patients who are infected—only those who have been exposed, which is virtually all of us. The American Academy of Allergy and Immunology issued a position paper stating that "the concept (of a yeast connection) is speculative and unproven . . . elements of the proposed treatment program are potentially dangerous."

MERCURY AMALGAMS

The use of mercury-silver amalgam fillings in the mouth has been held to produce chronic fatigue, headaches, cognitive dysfunction, and muscle and joint aches. Although the American Dental Association considers mercury amalgams to be a safe, effective method of tooth restoration, there may be an extremely small group of patients who are sensitive to this product. When patients with fibromyalgia raise this question, I reply that in 20 years of practice only 1 patient of mine (out of 12,000 seen) has had all symptoms disappear with the removal of mercury amalgam fillings.

INTERSTITIAL CYSTITIS

Interstitial cystitis is listed as a controversial condition because of its lack of a clear-cut definition. Classic interstitial cystitis is defined as pain, frequency, and urinary urgency in a patient with negative urine cultures. Cystoscopy reveals inflammation, blood, and frequently scarring when biopsy samples are viewed under the microscope. The bladder muscle wall can be thick, but the lining mucosa is friable and thin. Classic interstitial cystitis is seen in autoimmune diseases (especially lupus), after radiation therapy, and in patients who had chronic bladder infections in the past.

Unfortunately, some practitioners (particularly non-urologists) term what we call female urethral syndrome (see Chapter 13) interstitial cystitis; others use the term loosely on the basis of the above-listed symptoms without cystoscopic confirmation. Recent studies have shown that a type of white blood cell known as a *mast cell* is present in large numbers at the nerve endings in interstitial cystitis patients. The bladder wall also has high levels of substance P. An increased percentage of patients who fall into the categories listed in this paragraph have fibromyalgia.

SUMMING UP

If you have been diagnosed as having multiple chemical sensitivity syndrome, Gulf War syndrome, siliconosis, a leaky gut with or without yeast infection, heavy metal toxicity, or interstitial cystitis, be aware that these diagnoses are controversial and may not truly exist. Before initiating expensive, time-consuming, toxic, or lifestyle-altering therapies that are unproven, make sure that your treating physicians agree on the best course of action to take. Or at least, look before you leap!

Part V
THE EVALUATION OF FIBROMYALGIA PATIENTS

Patients with fibromyalgia-related symptoms may consult a variety of health care professionals and physicians in all specialties. This part reviews what patients and doctors look for, what tests are ordered, and how they are interpreted. How can a doctor be sure that the diagnosis is correct? Is another diagnosis being missed? And finally, is it really all in one's head?

15

What Happens at a Fibromyalgia Consultation?

We don't believe in rheumatism and true love until after the first attack.

Marie von Ebner-Eschenbach (1830–1916)

Fibromyalgia is usually a diagnosis of exclusion. Often poorly understood by some primary care physicians, the diagnosis of fibromyalgia is often delayed. In one survey, the diagnosis was made only after patients saw a mean of 3.5 doctors. This chapter will take you through the workup that establishes the definitive diagnosis and eliminates other possible explanations for the patient's complaints.

WHO SHOULD BE THE FIBROMYALGIA CONSULTANT AND HOW CAN THE PATIENT PREPARE FOR THE VISIT?

Doctors who diagnose and treat fibromyalgia often cross specialty lines. Although rheumatologists tend to regard fibromyalgia as residing within their bailiwick, there are too few of us to handle all the needs of the 6 million fibromyalgia sufferers. The 5000 rheumatologists in the United States are internal medicine subspecialists. A total of 80,000 doctors practice primary care internal medicine in the United States, and an additional 80,000 general or family practitioners are the front-line doctors for most patients. These physicians may suspect fibromyalgia and consult a rheumatologist to confirm the diagnosis. In complicated cases, the rheumatologist can take over the management of the condition. Orthopedists, neurosurgeons, and neurologists frequently diagnose fibromyalgia but generally refer patients to rheumatologists or internists for treatment. Rheumatologists may refer patients to physical medicine specialists or pain management centers when their approaches do not bear fruit.

Suppose that you are suspected of having fibromyalgia, and a primary care physician has referred you to a fibromyalgia consultant (usually a rheumatologist but sometimes an internist, physiatrist, neurologist, orthopedist, or osteopath) to confirm the diagnosis and make management suggestions. Is any sort of advanced preparation advisable? Yes. Bring copies of outside records and previous test results or workups to the consultant. If you have more than a few com-

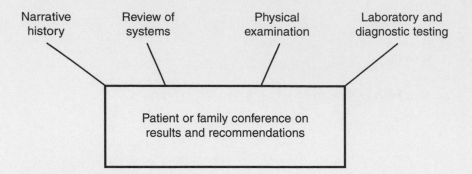

Fig. 18 *The fibromyalgia consultation. (From D. J. Wallace,* The Lupus Book. *New York: Oxford University Press, 1995, p. 123; reprinted with permission)*

plaints or are taking more than a few medications, a summary list is useful. The evaluation will consist of a history, physical examination, diagnostic laboratory tests, and possibly imaging studies (X-rays, scans, etc.). Once all the observations and test results are in, the doctor will discuss the findings with you—perhaps at the time of the visit, by telephone after the initial meeting, or in a follow-up visit. The consultation process is illustrated in Figure 18.

DR. WALLACE'S FIBROMYALGIA CONSULTATION: PATIENT INTERVIEW

I begin by asking why the patient has come in and how he or she feels. Once I've heard the patient's symptoms and history, I conduct a review of systems. As many as 100 questions can be asked as part of this screening process. Positive responses may lead to an additional set of queries that clarify symptoms in a given area, such as how long the complaint has been present, whether it is constant or intermittent, what time of day it is present, what makes it better or worse, how it has been diagnostically evaluated and treated in the past, and its current status.

I ask the patient about allergies and about family members' history of rheumatic disease or other diseases. Other relevant facts include possible occupational exposure to allergic or toxic substances, a detailed description of what his or her body does during the day, how much and what exercise or activities are performed, educational attainment, and with whom the patient lives. Unusual childhood diseases also are explored, as well as tobacco or alcohol use and abuse, immunizations, previous hospitalizations and surgeries, past and present prescriptions, and frequency of use of over-the-counter medications. These questions also provide the basis of a psychosocial profile, which may be important in developing a productive doctor-patient relationship.

The internal medicine/rheumatic review of systems covers these categories:

1. *Constitutional symptoms*, such as fevers, malaise, weight loss, or swollen glands, are dealt with first. They refer to the patient's overall state and how he or she feels. This is followed by an organ system review that goes from head to toes.

2. The *head and neck* review includes inquiries about cataracts, glaucoma, dry eyes, dry mouth, eye pain, jaw pain, double vision, loss of vision, iritis, conjunctivitis, ringing in the ears, loss of hearing, frequent ear infections, frequent nosebleeds, smell abnormalities, frequent sinus infections, sores in the nose or mouth, dental problems, or swollen glands in the neck.

3. The *cardiopulmonary* system is covered next. I ask about asthma, bronchitis, emphysema, tuberculosis, pleurisy (pain on taking a deep breath), shortness of breath, pneumonia, high blood pressure, chest pains, rheumatic fever, heart murmur, heart attack, palpitations, and irregular heartbeat.

4. The *gastrointestinal* system review includes an effort to find any evidence of swallowing difficulties, severe nausea or vomiting, diarrhea, constipation, unusual eating habits, hepatitis, bloating, flatulence, ulcers, gallstones, blood in stool or vomit, diverticulitis, colitis, or pancreatitis.

5. The *genitourinary* area should be approached in a respectful, sensitive way. In addition to inquiring about frequent bladder infections, kidney stones, prostate problems, or blood or protein in the urine, I review the obstetrical history, breast disorders, and menstrual problems.

6. Next, the *hematologic* and *immune* factors that the patient may be aware of include how easily he or she bruises, anemia, low white blood cell or platelet counts, and frequent infections.

7. A *neuropsychiatric* history takes into account headaches, seizures, numbness or tingling, fainting, psychiatric or antidepressant interventions, substance abuse, difficulty sleeping, and cognitive dysfunction. If it is relevant and I feel comfortable approaching the subject, sexual dysfunction, a history of sexual abuse, domestic violence, or physical abuse may be reviewed. This may also be the time to inquire about blood transfusions or even AIDS risk factors.

8. *Musculoskeletal* concerns involve a history of joint pain, stiffness, gout, muscle pains, or weakness and better characterization of the complaints of fibromyalgia.

9. The *endocrine* system review includes questions about thyroid disease, diabetes, and high cholesterol level.

10. The *vascular* history may uncover prior episodes of phlebitis, clots, swelling, fluid retention, strokes, or Raynaud's phenomenon (fingers turning different colors in cold weather).

11. Finally, the *skin* is discussed. Evidence of sun sensitivity, hair loss, mouth sores, rashes, psoriasis, eczema, or changes in skin coloring is reviewed carefully.

In concluding the history taking, I always ask the patient whether there is anything I should know that was not covered. One of my mentors, Edmund Dubois, devoted his rheumatology textbook to "the patients, from whom we have learned." Physicians become better doctors when they listen to what patients have to say about things that the doctor may not have brought up. Occasionally, the patient mentions something in a casual conversation that turns out to be quite important in shedding light on his or her health problems.

THE PHYSICAL EXAMINATION

The history and review of systems elucidate what physicians call *symptoms*; a physical examination reveals *signs*. Four methods known as *inspection* (looking at an area), *palpation* (feeling an area), *percussion* (gentle knocking against a surface such as the lung or liver to detect fullness or size), and *auscultation* (listening with a stethoscope to the heart, chest, carotid artery, etc.) are employed during the complete physical. Patients are evaluated from head to toe.

First, *vital signs* are checked to ascertain weight, pulse, respirations, blood pressure, and temperature. The *head and neck* exam includes evaluation of the pupils' response to light, eye movements, cataracts, and vessels of the eye. The ear exam searches for obstruction and inflammation. The oral cavity is screened for sores, poor dental hygiene, and dryness. I palpate the thyroid and the glands of the neck and also listen to the neck for abnormal murmurs or sounds (carotid artery bruits). The *chest* examination consists of inspection (e.g., for postural abnormalities), palpation for chest wall tenderness, percussion to detect fluid in the lungs, and auscultation (e.g., to rule out asthma or pneumonia). The *heart* is checked for murmurs, clicks, or irregular beats. The *abdomen* is inspected for obesity, distention, or scars; palpated for pain or hernia; percussed to assess the size of the liver and spleen; and auscultated to rule out any obstruction or vascular sounds. This is followed by an *extremity* evaluation, which includes looking for swelling, color changes, inflamed joints, and deformities. Specific maneuvers allow me to assess range of motion, muscle strength, pulses, muscle tone, and fibromyalgia tender points. If indicated, a genitourinary evaluation is done. It includes a breast examination, rectal evaluation, and pelvic examination (in women a Pap smear and in men a prostate exam). In rheumatology, a genitourinary exam is necessary only if the patient has complaints relevant to these areas and no other physician has recently performed one. A *neurobehavioral* assessment reflecting change in mental status is usually conducted as part of the ongoing conversation; neurologic deficits can be detected by observing the patient for tremor, gait abnormalities, or abnormal sensation, movements, or reflexes. Finally, the *skin* is examined for rashes, pigment changes, tattoos, hair loss, Raynaud's phenomenon, and skin breakdown or ulcerations.

The physical examination may include other steps as well, depending upon the problem reported and the nature of the consultation. A thorough physical examination is usually conducted after a detailed interview and allows me to order appropriate tests.

MUST BLOOD BE DRAWN OR URINE EXAMINED?

A history and physical examination may suggest the diagnosis of fibromyalgia, but in order to make sure that other disorders with complaints and physical findings similar to those of fibromyalgia are not present, it is necessary to perform blood laboratory tests.

When a patient arrives at an internist's or family practitioner's office for a general medical evaluation, it usually includes what doctors refer to as *screening laboratory tests*. In other words, by obtaining a blood count, urine test, and blood chemistry panel, abnormalities can be detected in 90 percent of individuals with serious medical problems. All the tests listed below are inexpensive and mostly automated; they can be performed within hours and do not require special expertise. Most large medical offices are equipped to perform these tests on the premises. In fibromyalgia the tests are almost always normal.

A *complete blood count* (*CBC*) analyzes your red blood cells, white blood cells, and platelets (which are responsible for clotting). The CBC screens for anemia, infections, risk factors for infection, and bleeding disorders. *Blood chemistry* panels consist of anywhere from 7 to 25 tests that evaluate a variety of parameters, including blood sugar, kidney function (blood urea nitrogen [BUN], creatinine), liver function (aspartate aminotransferase [AST], alanine aminotransferase [ALT], bilirubin, alkaline phosphatase, gamma glutamyltransferase [GGT]), electrolytes (sodium, potassium, chloride, bicarbonate, calcium, phosphorus, magnesium), lipids or fats (cholesterol, triglycerides, high density lipoprotein [HDL], low density lipoprotein [LDL]), proteins (albumin, total protein), thyroid function (triiodothyronine [T_3], thyroxine [T_4], thyroid-stimulating hormone [TSH]), and gout (uric acid). Occasionally chemistry panels include additional studies (amylase for pancreatic function, lactic dehydrogenase [LDH] for red blood cell breakdown, iron or vitamin B_{12} levels), which are also inexpensive and can be added upon request. Other inexpensive blood tests that may be asked for include a creatine phosphokinase (CPK) to rule out muscle inflammation, a Westergren sedimentation rate or C-reactive protein test to rule out inflammation in the bloodstream or tissues, and tests for clotting time (prothrombin time [PT], partial thromboplastin time [PTT], bleeding time). A *urinalysis* is a useful screen for kidney disease, kidney stones, urinary tract infections, and other conditions.

WHEN ARE IMAGING STUDIES, ELECTRICAL EVALUATIONS, AND SPECIALIZED BLOOD TESTS REQUESTED?

When evaluating a potential fibromyalgia patient, I usually obtain a chest X-ray and ECG of the heart if one has not been done recently. These are also inexpensive and safe procedures that rule out potentially important causes of chest area pains, palpitations, and shortness of breath.

In certain circumstances, additional blood testing may be useful. Autoimmune blood tests consisting of an ANA or rheumatoid factor screen for systemic lupus and rheumatoid arthritis may be necessary. If these tests are positive, as they are in a small number of fibromyalgia patients, specific additional ANA panels can be obtained to confirm the diagnosis. Fibromyalgia patients frequently complain of numbness, tingling, and burning. The doctor may want to get X-rays (and, if abnormal, an MRI or computed tomography [CT] scan) of the neck or low back to make sure that a bone spur or herniated disc is not causing these symptoms. An EMG can also diagnose herniated discs or indicate if numbness is from carpal tunnel syndrome, diabetes, or an inflammatory process. In difficult cases, a spinal X-ray performed after injecting dye into the spinal column, known as a *myelogram*, usually determines if a herniated disc is present. Bone scans can look for tumors or inflammation. Sleep EEGs (polysomnography) may be ordered if it is important to document a physiologic basis for complaints of unrefreshing sleep.

There are additional blood tests, imaging, and electrical studies that are inexpensive and useful and may be appropriate in specific situations. Some of them are reviewed in the next chapter.

ARE THERE UNPROVEN DIAGNOSTIC TESTS?

Occasionally, doctors order tests that are not necessary and others that have no known value. Unproven testing consists of procedures that needlessly run up the bill, are never helpful in the diagnosis and/or treatment of the patient, are not covered by insurance companies, and are considered invalid by most doctors. Few of these studies will change anything a knowledgeable doctor would do for the patient. In patients with probable primary fibromyalgia, I see no reason to order T- and B-cell counts with lymphocyte subsets; tests for mitogenic stimulation; yeast antibody levels; nail, hair, or body chemical analysis; cytotoxic testing; skin endpoint titration; provocation-neutralization testing; cytokine and cytokine receptor assays; or a food immune complex assay. Check out a doctor's credentials before taking the plunge. Call your local hospital, medical association, or university. Is the doctor board certified by a specialty recognized by the American College of Physicians or the American Board of Medical Specialties?

SUMMING UP

If a primary care doctor has referred a patient to a qualified specialist to confirm a diagnosis or make suggestions on how to manage fibromyalgia, it's helpful for the patient to be organized, direct, and have easy-to-digest summaries of past and present medical complaints, prior blood tests, imaging or electrical evaluations, and treatments. The specialist will perform a comprehensive evaluation, which should provide the primary care doctor with the consultation or information needed to assure patients the highest quality care.

16

Are You Sure It's Really Fibromyalgia?

Ever since I have been ill, I have longed and longed for some palpable disease, no matter how conventionally dreadful a label it might have, but I was always driven back to stagger alone under the monstrous mass of subjective sensations, which that sympathetic being "The Medicine Man" had no higher inspiration than to assure me I was personally responsible for, washing his hands of me with a graceful complacency.
                    Alice James (1848–1892), *The Diary of Alice James*

A week doesn't go by without a patient wanting my reassurance that he or she is not seriously ill or making it all up. "Are you just telling me it's fibromyalgia because you don't want me to be upset?" "A friend of mine told me that fibromyalgia is a 'garbage can' diagnosis that doctors give when they don't know what you have." These are frequent remarks or queries. How is your doctor really sure that something is not being missed? This chapter reviews some diseases with features that can overlap with or be mistaken for fibromyalgia.

FIBROMYALGIA CAN BE PART OF OTHER DISEASES

Fibromyalgia can seem to be working in concert with other diseases. For example, untreated inflammation associated with an autoimmune disease (such as rheumatoid arthritis or systemic lupus erythematosus), other forms of inflammatory arthritis (such as ankylosing spondylitis), or a chest disease known as *sarcoidosis* are associated with coexisting fibromyalgia. Withdrawal from or tapering of medications such as corticosteroids typically precipitates or aggravates fibromyalgia.

SOME DISORDERS CAN MIMIC OR INTERACT WITH FIBROMYALGIA

Many disorders interact with or can be mistaken for fibromyalgia. They are reviewed here, as well as in other parts of this book, and listed in Table 9.

Table 9. *Common disorders that can mimic fibromyalgia*

Hormonal imbalances
   Menstrual disorders
   Low thyroid, high parathyroid levels
   Pregnancy
   Adrenal insufficiency
   Diabetes
   Menopause
Infections
   Bacteria
   Viruses
   Fungi
   Parasites
Musculoskeletal or autoimmune disorders
   Rheumatoid arthritis
   Ankylosing spondylitis in females
   Seronegative spondyloarthropathies
   Lyme disease
   Systemic lupus erythematosus
   Palindromic rheumatism
   Inflammatory bowel disease
   Polymyalgia rheumatica
Neurologic disease
   Multiple sclerosis
   Myasthenia gravis
Malignancy
Substance abuse
Malnutrition
Primary psychiatric disorders
Allergies

Hormonal imbalances

Linda was not herself. Over a period of several months, she found it increasingly difficult to make it through the day. Her muscles started to ache, she gained 15 pounds while on the same diet, found it difficult to tolerate cold weather, and her voice became husky. Dr. Bridges did a complete blood count and a blood panel that was normal. He was impressed with her muscle aches and diagnosed her as having fibromyalgia. When Dr. White saw Linda in a rheumatology consultation, certain things did not fit. Weight gain, a hoarse voice, and cold intolerance of recent onset are not typical features of fibromyalgia, so she obtained additional tests which included a complete thyroid panel (triiodothyronine [T_3], thyroxine [T_4], thyroid-stimulating hormone [TSH]). Although the T_3 and T_4 levels were normal (as they had been with Dr. Bridges), the TSH (which was not part of Dr. Bridges's panel) was quite high, indicating hypothyroidism. Linda was started on thyroid replacement therapy and was back to herself within a few weeks.

Low *thyroid* levels, or *hypothyroidism* can be mistaken for fibromyalgia. Blood T_3, T_4, and TSH tests readily and inexpensively differentiate these disorders. *Parathyroid tumors* or adenomas raise blood calcium levels and cause aching, weakness, and palpitations. The parathyroid gland overlies the thyroid, and disorders of this gland are detected by measuring calcium, phosphorus, and parathormone blood levels. *Adrenal glands* overlie the kidney and make cortisone. Adrenal insufficiency (Addison's disease) or adrenal overactivity (Cushing's disease) can modulate fibromyalgia symptoms. *Diabetics* with peripheral nerve disease complain of numbness and tingling. If their sugar level is too high or too low, they complain of fatigue, palpitations, and weakness.

Hormonal disorders produce fatigue, aching and weakness. *Premenstrual syndrome (PMS)* frequently aggravates fibromyalgia symptoms. *Menopause* can improve fibromyalgia, but early menopausal symptoms can mimic and aggravate the syndrome. Irregular periods, use of birth control pills, and painful periods may produce symptoms of bloating, fatigue, and aching. It is also important to make sure that new fibromyalgia-like symptoms are not in fact an early *pregnancy*.

Infections

Bacteria, viruses, fungi, parasites, and other microbes infect the body and produce a variety of systemic reactions, including fatigue, malaise, fevers, swollen glands, rashes, joint pain, shortness of breath, abdominal pain, and difficulty thinking clearly. Infections and fibromyalgia can interact in three different ways: postinfectious fatigue syndromes can cause fibromyalgia and chronic fatigue syndrome, fibromyalgia may be mistaken for infection and vice versa, and infections can aggravate fibromyalgia.

A doctor can screen for infections with the workup reviewed in the previous chapter but may need additional tests. These may include cultures of blood, urine, sputum, stool, bone marrow, skin lesions, spinal fluid, pleural fluid, or whatever bodily tissues are accessible, and serum antibody levels to organisms to ascertain prior or current exposure. Sometimes, doctors perform skin tests (such as a tuberculosis skin test) or order scans to identify infected areas. Infections should be promptly identified and treated.

Musculoskeletal disorders

As mentioned earlier, 7–22 percent of patients with autoimmune diseases have secondary fibromyalgia and may be mistakenly diagnosed as having the syndrome. Early *rheumatoid arthritis* sometimes appears fibromyalgia-like before it settles in the hands and feet and causes joint swelling. *Systemic lupus erythematosus* is commonly misdiagnosed as fibromyalgia because overlapping fatigue, aching, and cognitive impairment symptoms can be confusing. Ten million Americans have a positive ANA, which is almost always seen in lupus, but only 1 million Americans have lupus. Therefore, patients who present to a rheumatologist with a positive ANA and nonspecific symptoms often go through a workup to rule out lupus, which may include obtaining muscle enzymes, inflammatory indices such as sedimentation rate, skin biopsy specimens, bone scans, and detailed autoantibody blood testing. *Polymyositis* is an inflammatory muscle disease differentiated from fibromyalgia by elevation of the muscle enzyme creatine phosphokinase in blood testing.

Rheumatoid variants such as *ankylosing spondylitis, psoriatic arthritis, arthritis of inflammatory bowel disease,* and *Reiter's syndrome* may be hard to distinguish from fibromyalgia since they are often only intermittently inflammatory. Many rheumatoid variant patients have a positive blood test for a marker known as HLA-B27. *Palindromic rheumatism* presents as a pre-rheumatoid arthritis, pre-lupus-like condition, with infrequent physical findings of joint swelling and symptoms of aching and fatigue. *Polymyalgia rheumatica* is seen in older patients who have aching in their shoulder and hip areas; it is usually easy to differentiate from fibromyalgia since the blood sedimentation rate is elevated.

Hypermobility syndromes and *work overuse syndromes* may be misdiagnosed as fibromyalgia but are associated with regional myofascial syndromes, as are *osteoarthritis, spinal stenosis*, and *disc problems* in the cervical and lumbar spines. Most people in their 40s and 50s have nonspecific abnormalities on X-rays or CT or MRI scans, and sometimes low back pain or neck pain is interpreted as a herniated disc when it is really due to fibromyalgia.

Neurologic disease

Tina was a tireless housewife who always did three things at once. One day, she dropped the bag she was carrying from the car while experiencing a "weak spell." Over the following weeks, Tina noticed some numbness and tingling in her legs that her husband thought could be a herniated disc from her vigorous workout. Her family doctor was not sure what the problem was and made an offhand remark that it could be due to a flu or a type of fibromyalgia. Over the next week, Tina became unsteady as she walked and complained of being dizzy. An MRI scan of her brain was diagnostic for multiple sclerosis, and she was referred to a neurologist for treatment.

Patients with early forms of *multiple sclerosis* and *myasthenia gravis* complain of numbness, aching, fatigue, weakness, and difficulty thinking clearly without dramatic physical findings. Unlike fibromyalgia, multiple sclerosis is characterized by MRI and spinal fluid abnormalities, and myasthenia gravis is marked by abnormal electrical studies and positive antibody tests. To further confuse the issue, secondary fibromyalgia accompanies neurologic disease in up to 20 percent of these patients. Primary muscle or nerve disorders associated with complaints of numbness, tingling, or burning can be differentiated from fibromyalgia by EMG and nerve conduction studies, as well as by various forms of spinal imaging. Nerve or muscle biopsies are occasionally recommended to clarify the diagnosis.

Malignancies

Patients with cancer make a variety of extra chemicals, many of which cause systemic symptoms, including fatigue, aching, and weakness, that resemble fibromyalgia complaints. These *paraneoplastic* features of a tumor usually disappear with treatment including chemotherapy, radiation therapy, and surgery. Steroids frequently are used along with chemotherapy, and disease onset and/or changes can produce fibromyalgia. Selected drugs used to treat cancer, such as *alpha-interferon* (for leukemia) or *interleukin-2* (e.g., for melanoma or kidney cancer) may induce fibromyalgia-like symptoms that last for weeks to months. Healthy-appearing young women with early stages of *Hodgkin's disease* and other *lymphomas* initially have been diagnosed incorrectly as having fibromyalgia.

Substance abuse and malnutrition

Things were not going well for Kelly. Although her fibromyalgia was under fair control, Kelly always seemed tired. She never appeared to eat regularly, and her weight dropped below 100 pounds. Kelly was becoming an alcoholic. When the judge cut her divorce payments by half and her children left for college, Kelly advanced from being a social drinker at night to consuming cocktails whenever she could. It took a while for her friends to catch on. Kelly was very good at hiding her habit and drank six to eight cups of coffee or cola drinks a day. She stole diet pills from her friends' medicine cabinets to give her more energy. Kelly's self-destructive actions persisted until her three best friends took her to Spa Ranch near Death Valley, California, for a weekend. Kelly promptly convulsed from alcohol withdrawal and was cut off from her caffeine and stimulants. At the nearby community hospital, Kelly's fibromyalgia pain was excruciating. After she returned home, her family physician helped her enter the Alcoholics Anonymous program, and she graduated successfully from the 12-step program. Her muscles now rarely hurt, and she is receiving counseling.

Our society provides many means—legal and otherwise—to obtain agents that can produce or alleviate fatigue. Caffeine is an addictive chemical in coffee, tea, headache formulas (e.g., Excedrin, Fiorinal), and cola beverages that can increase the heart rate. People who are dependent on caffeine develop fatigue and palpitations or withdrawal symptoms when they are deprived of it for a day or two. Many of these individuals take diet pills or "uppers" to manage fatigue, which can also lead to appetite loss, weight loss, and malnutrition.

The number of patients who complain of profound fatigue and do not realize (or deny) that it could be due to taking high doses of prescription painkillers such as Vicodin, codeine, Darvon, or Percocet is amazing. Alcohol, cocaine, and heroin abuse are common causes of fatigue, but dependence on pain medicine is very common. Sudden withdrawal of any of these substances is associated with pain amplification.

FIBROMYALGIA CAN APPEAR DIFFERENT IN DIFFERENT AGE GROUPS

When fibromyalgia appears in very young and elderly patients, it is not only uncommon but presents differently than expected. New-onset fibromyalgia in these age groups can be very difficult to diagnose.

Fibromyalgia in childhood and adolescence

Diana was every mother's dream. A 14-year-old girl from a comfortable middle-class family, she was an honor student, star of the volleyball team, and president of her church youth group. Diana never complained, was very serious, spent more time on her homework assignments than was necessary, and sometimes had difficulty relaxing. While serving at the volleyball championship, she felt a pop in her right shoulder, which swelled up a few hours later. The pain and swelling were not only uncomfortable but also very upsetting. Over the following weeks, Diana's shoulder seemed frozen and immovable and both of her hands became puffy, especially on the right. Although the initial mechanical problem in her right shoulder slowly healed with physical therapy. Diana became very tired, achy, and depressed, had difficulty sleeping, and became aware of numerous tender points. A pediatric rheumatologist diagnosed her as having juvenile fibromyalgia with reflex sympathetic dystrophy. Diana was given ibuprofen and a few steroid injections into her shoulder, and a vigorous rehabilitation program was prescribed. Although the therapy was quite painful at first, Diana slowly responded to it. A psychologist working with the rehabilitation center taught her biofeedback, yoga, and relaxation techniques. Her perfectionistic tendencies were redirected in a more socially useful direction.

Whereas fibromyalgia is present in 2 percent of adults and is the 3rd or 4th most common reason for seeking a rheumatology consultation, it is the 12th most common reason for seeking a pediatric rheumatology evaluation. Pediatric rheumatologists see a new child or adolescent with fibromyalgia just a few times a year. There are probably fewer than 10,000 children in the United States with the syndrome, 90 percent of whom are adolescents. This has led some investigators to speculate that a hormonal connection may be very important. In addition to its relative rarity, preadult fibromyalgia is different from adult fibromyalgia. How so? In two ways: reflex sympathetic dystrophy (RSD) and a typical psychiatric profile.

Few centers have much experience with childhood fibromyalgia, but studies from Children's Hospital of Los Angeles suggest that a subset of adolescents with fibromyalgia fit a specific profile. An example could be a 10- to 15-year old girl who has grown up as a "perfect, model" child, never complains, and has perfectionistic tendencies and excellent grades in school. A seemingly trivial sports injury or emotional event can be followed by widespread pain and fatigue. Additionally, reflex sympathetic dystrophy with swelling of both upper extremities (more severe on one side than on the other), inability to move an arm or shoulder, and mottling changes in the skin is often present. RSD is found in 1–10 percent of adult fibromyalgia patients but is seen in 20–80 percent of adolescents. Adolescents with severe growing pains, disturbed sleep, irritable colon, attention deficit, and hypermobile (very limber) joints frequently develop full-blown fibromyalgia in adulthood.

Unlike adult fibromyalgia, the juvenile syndrome responds only minimally to tricyclic antidepressants and pain medication. The best results correlate with intensive, vigorous physical therapy and exercise, steroid injections to affected areas or intermittent courses of oral steroids, and psychological support. Even though the presentation of fibromyalgia in young people is more severe than in adults, children and adolescents have a better prognosis than many adults. If the treatment program outlined above is aggressively pursued, 80 percent of young patients have substantial resolution of the syndrome within 2–3 years.

Fibromyalgia in the elderly

Wilma starting fading after her 70th birthday. She began complaining of aching in her middle and upper back areas, in addition to stiffness in her wrists and hands. Wilma's doctor performed blood tests that showed a slightly elevated sedimentation rate, which could signify inflammation. Dr. Lear was not sure whether this was polymyalgia rheumatica, a common joint disease among senior citizens, or early rheumatoid arthritis. Wilma also had fatigue, tension headaches, and difficulty sleeping. However, Dr. Lear seemed so busy and rushed that she was too intimidated to take up his valuable time by reporting these symptoms, which she thought were less important. Wilma was given low-dose prednisone, 10 mg a day, which helped greatly during the first week. Over the following month, her symptoms worsened and Wilma became anxious and panicky. Dr. Lear referred her to Dr. Green, who took a more detailed history. In the last year Wilma had lost her son, been involved in an automobile accident, and caught a bad flu; her best friend had had a serious stroke. Dr. Green diagnosed her as having fibromyalgia, tapered her steroids, referred her to a gerontology patient support center, and prescribed low-dose bedtime nortriptyline (Pamelor), an antidepressant that promotes restful sleep.

As patients with long-standing fibromyalgia age, the syndrome usually persists. Many female patients report that menopause modestly decreases their symptoms. But can people over the age of 65 develop fibromyalgia-like symptoms? Since this is an unusual event, the differential diagnosis reviewed earlier in this chapter should be considered. This applies especially to hypothyroidism, Sjogren's syndrome (dry eyes, dry mouth, aching, and fatigue), rheumatoid arthritis, occult malignancy, and polymyalgia rheumatica. A normal sedimentation rate, negative ANA, negative rheumatoid factor, and normal TSH (thyroid test) usually allow doctors to make a definitive diagnosis of fibromyalgia. Studies of patients with older-onset fibromyalgia show fewer functional symptoms such as anxiety, stress, or unrefreshed sleep and more musculoskeletal complaints than their younger counterparts. Polymyalgia rheumatica is far more common than late-onset fibromyalgia. It presents with aching in the upper back, neck, buttocks, or thighs, along with a markedly elevated sedimentation rate. Many healthy older people have modestly elevated sedimentation rates. As a consequence, up to 40 percent of late-onset fibromyalgia patients in one survey were given corticosteroids before a correct diagnosis was made. Older-onset fibromyalgia is managed the same way as in younger adults. Finally, joint and muscle aches can be symptomatic of primary depression; this possibility always warrants careful consideration.

DEAR DOCTOR: THINK OF FIBROMYALGIA

Make no mistake about it. Fibromyalgia will never be diagnosed unless a doctor considers it to be a diagnostic possibility. Many doctors were trained before accepted definitions and criteria for the syndrome were established. We have seen many patients who had cancer workups, expensive MRI and CT scans, adrenal evaluations, and even surgical procedures when a better-focused workup would have revealed the real problem. Managed care has caused many doctors to think twice before ordering these expensive studies or asking for help from a consultant. "Megaworkups" will decrease over the next few years as our health care environment changes and continuing medical education for physicians becomes more widespread.

SUMMING UP

Fibromyalgia is a diagnosis of exclusion. Serious and treatable disorders with overlapping symptoms and signs should be ruled out before patients are convinced and the doctor feels comfortable with the diagnosis. If a patient has fibromyalgia secondary to one of several disorders, it won't get better until the primary or underlying disease is addressed. Doctors try their best, but the patient's symptoms, signs, and physical findings can be subtle and don't always lead directly to a diagnosis of fibromyalgia.

17

I'm Not Crazy!

*A bodily disease, which we look upon as whole and entire
within itself, may, after all, be but a symptom of some ailment
in the spiritual part.*

Nathaniel Hawthorne (1804–1864)

"You look fine, and I can't find anything wrong with you. Maybe you're just depressed or stressed out." Nearly all of my patients have heard this before. And they start to wonder: Am I really crazy? How could it all be in my mind? This chapter will summarize the small number of behavioral surveys that rheumatologists and psychiatrists have performed on fibromyalgia patients. The treatment of fibromyalgia will be reviewed in Parts VI and VII.

Why are there so few studies that we can rely upon? First, most research is conducted at university medical centers, where fibromyalgia patients tend to be more symptomatic and have not responded to interventions by community physicians. Second, depression itself is associated with high rates of musculoskeletal pain. Also, few people have had comprehensive psychological evaluations *before* they became ill that can be used for comparison. Finally, instruments of psychological assessment were devised before we knew what fibromyalgia was, and popular tests such as the Minnesota Multiphasic Personality Inventory (MMPI) cannot distinguish between pain from a disease and pain from depression.

DO I HURT BECAUSE I'M DEPRESSED OR
AM I DEPRESSED BECAUSE I HURT?

Is fibromyalgia a manifestation of depression or the reverse? About 20 well-designed studies have addressed this issue. They all used different methods, populations, ethnic groupings, referral sources, and geographical distributions. In any case, the results were reasonably similar. On average, these studies showed that about 18 percent of fibromyalgia patients have evidence of a major depression at any office visit and 58 percent have a history of major depression in their lifetime. What does this mean? *At any point in time, the overwhelming majority of fibromyalgia patients are not seriously depressed.* And if they are depressed, it's usually because they do not feel well. This condition is called *reactive depression* and is reversible with treatment, as opposed to *endogenous depres-*

sion, which is caused by chemical imbalances and is much harder to treat. A well-designed study of depressed patients demonstrated that fewer than 10 percent had two or more tender points.

ARE THERE HISTORICAL BEHAVIORAL FACTORS THAT ARE MORE COMMON IN FIBROMYALGIA PATIENTS THAN IN THOSE WITHOUT THE DISORDER?

Certain life events or historical factors are statistically present more often in fibromyalgia patients than in those without the disorder. This does not mean that more than a minority of patients have had these problems. Statistical methods have allowed us to do *case control studies*, in which each fibromyalgia patient is matched with a person without fibromyalgia who is of the same age, race, and sex. Some case control studies also match geographic locations, educational backgrounds, socioeconomic status, and other factors. One popular method is for each patient in a study to pick a healthy friend as the control. Mathematical formulas allow surveyors to devise a *relative risk* or *odds ratio*. For example, a survey might determine in a case controlled fashion that a patient is twice as likely to have a family history of alcoholism or cancer as a friend with a relative risk of 2.0, or 2 to 1. This, for example, makes the odds twice as likely that fibromyalgia patients will have these features.

A handful of controversial studies conducted in the last few years show that fibromyalgia patients have a significantly increased risk of having a history of sexual, physical, or drug abuse, eating disorders, mood disorders, manic-depression (bipolar disease), obsessive-compulsive disorder, attention deficit disorder, phobias (unrealistic fears), panic, anxiety, somatization, and a family history of depression or alcoholism. They also show that fibromyalgia patients cope less well with daily problems than others and are more susceptible to psychological stress. We have already shown that psychological stress can lower the pain threshold. The studies also suggest that there is more *alexithymia,* a long-standing personality disorder with generalized and localized complaints in individuals who cannot express their underlying psychological conflicts. As a consequence, some behavioral experts have proposed that fibromyalgia is an *affective spectrum disorder* in which a primary psychiatric disorder with a possibly inherited abnormality leads to pain amplification and fibromyalgia-related complaints.

WHAT'S WRONG WITH THE AFFECTIVE SPECTRUM MODEL OF FIBROMYALGIA?

These studies have promoted an intense debate among fibromyalgia experts as to whether fibromyalgia is a manifestation of a *psychological* disturbance or a *physiological* disorder of pain amplification. We strongly believe that the latter explanation is more accurate. Why do we feel so strongly? First, biochemical abnormalities (e.g., increased substance P level in spinal fluid) have been found in fibromyalgia that do not correlate with behavioral abnormalities. Second, fibromyalgia frequently occurs in conditions such as scoliosis, which have never been associated with any behavioral disorders. Third, all of the behavioral surveys supporting an affective spectrum disorder were performed at university medical centers and do not reflect what an internist or family physician sees in a community fibromyalgia population practice. For example, sexual abuse may be one of *many* triggers or aggravating factors of fibromyalgia syndrome, but it is seen in an extremely small number of patients with the disorder. For most patients followed in a community practice, the disease is not serious enough for them to be referred to a specialist. Specialists generally deal with more severe cases, which skews their study results. A recent study by Dr. Laurence Bradley at the University of Alabama has clearly proven this point.

ALPHABET SOUP: DSM-IV AND DSS

Many of us have some sort of doctrine that helps guide our actions. You might rely on the Holy Scriptures for advice. The Internal Revenue Service relies on the tax code, a rheumatologist on the ACR criteria, and psychiatrists on the DSM-IV. What is DSM-IV and why is it important? DSM-IV is the fourth revision of the *Diagnostic and Statistical Manual of Mental Disorders*. Since 1917, psychiatrists have tried their best to define and describe mental disorders according to the research and temperament of the times. Although subject to some political and social influences (e.g., whether or not homosexuality is a behavioral disorder has been debated for years; currently, it is not listed at all), DSM-IV carries immense weight in medical and legal circles.

Published in 1994, DSM-IV does not mention the word *fibromyalgia*, but in describing *undifferentiated somatization disorder* it does mention myofascial pain syndrome, chronic fatigue, neurasthenia, pain relating to the back or joints, and functional bowel complaints. Psychiatrists consider these complaints to be a disorder if there is no obvious medical explanation for the constellation of symptoms and signs. These symptoms and signs are real and cause significant impairment in social, occupational, and other important areas of functioning. Varying degrees of somatization syndromes are described, and many of the definitions do not apply to fibromyalgia. Although some investigators thought fibromyalgia was a somatization disorder in the 1970s and early 1980s, nearly all investigators today agree that it is not. The DSM-IV definition of somatization syndrome requires at least one pseudoneurologic symptom (such as saying "I can't see" or "My legs are paralyzed") that is clearly not part of fibromyalgia.

If an affective spectrum and a somatization model do not accurately fit fibromyalgia, what does? Dr. Muhammed Yunus has recognized that there are many

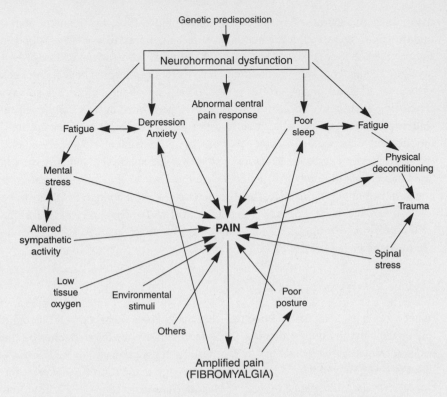

Fig. 19 *How chemicals associated with behavior biologically influence pain.*

overlapping features among fibromyalgia, migraine, irritable colon, and tension headaches, for example. He has proposed that fibromyalgia is a *dysregulation spectrum syndrome* (DSS). Excluding all psychiatric diagnoses, Dr. Yunus and many of his colleagues now feel that fibromyalgia should be studied using the biomedical model. While agreeing that DSS is influenced by factors that govern psychological behavior, such as personality, mood, and attitude, the DSS model stresses that neurotransmitters are capable of biologically altering pain perception. Figure 19 demonstrates some of these interactions.

ARE THERE OTHER DSM-IV DISORDERS THAT FIBROMYALGIA PATIENTS DO NOT HAVE AND THAT REQUIRE DIFFERENTIATION?

There are other conditions that some doctors confuse with fibromyalgia, and several surveys cited above show that patients generally do *not* have them. Some of these conditions are described below.

As of this writing, DSM-IV makes no accommodation for fibromyalgia. As the DSM committee becomes aware of rapid advances in the field, hopefully there will be a new category relating to DSS where biochemically mediated pain amplification influences behavior and physiologic responses.

Hypochondriasis

Hypochondriacs have an excessive fear of having a serious disease based on misinterpretation of one or more bodily symptoms and signs. They believe normal bodily sensations such as heartbeats and peristalsis represent a medical disorder. Nearly all fibromyalgia patients want to get well and accept reassurance that they are not seriously ill.

Hysteria (conversion reactions)

The psychiatric definition of hysteria differs from the common perception that these are individuals who are prone to ranting or raving. Hysterical patients complain of neurologic or body deficits that are not real and display a lack of concern (la belle indifference) or act blasé about them. These conversion reactions involve statements that they cannot see, hear, or talk, or are paralyzed. An example would be a soldier in battle who reports that he cannot move his legs. Some aspects of hysteria infrequently overlap with fibromyalgia, but hysteria is usually not associated with the syndrome.

Psychogenic rheumatism

Patients who claim that they "hurt all over" but lack fibromyalgia tender points and have changing stories with inappropriate or inconsistent responses have a *factitious disease* known as *psychogenic rheumatism*. These patients have serious emotional problems, and their complaints satisfy the psychological need for attention. Some are *psychotic*, or have lost touch with reality. Their stories make no biologic sense. The classic example is the patient who complains that "I hurt on the left side of my body, from the top of my head to the bottom of my toe." Anatomically, this is impossible since the nerve supply of these areas crosses the spinal cord at the neck and the head would hurt on the opposite side. Tender points are not found on examination, and no arthritis or muscle-focused therapies ever work. *Malingering*, or producing symptoms and signs for external gain, is not a feature of fibromyalgia.

Body dysmorphic disorder

Sometimes we encounter patients who are engrossed with themselves. They express excessive concern or fear of having a defect in appearance, a condition termed *body dysmorphic disorder* by DSM-IV. These patients obsess over every blemish or bruise. Studies have shown no correlation between this behavior pattern and fibromyalgia.

Obsessive-compulsive behavior

In the morning she was asked how she slept. "Oh terribly badly!" said the Princess. "I have scarcely shut my eyes the whole night. Heaven only knows what was in the bed, but I was lying on something hard, so that I am black and blue all over. . . ." Nobody but a real princess could be as sensitive as that. So the prince took her for his wife, for now he knew he had a real princess.

Hans Christian Andersen (1805–1875),
The Princess and the Pea, 1835

Many doctors think that most fibromyalgia patients have perfectionistic tendencies. After all, many new fibromyalgia patients came to us with a neatly typed, detailed medical history and list of complaints. *Obsessive-compulsive personality disorder,* consisting of a preoccupation with orderliness, perfectionism, and mental and interpersonal control at the expense of flexibility, openness, and efficiency, was found in the *affective spectrum* model of fibromyalgia, which we reject, but not in the *dysregulation spectrum syndrome* model, which we endorse. Perhaps our patients simply had been to so many doctors who did not believe their stories that they wanted to make sure they were better prepared for their next consultation and tried to report any symptoms, signs, or historical observations that could possibly be useful. The bottom line is that perfectionism as part of obsessive-compulsive personality disorder is not more common, but perfectionistic tendencies, as reviewed in Chapter 20, may be.

SUMMING UP

We prefer to view fibromyalgia in terms of a biomedical model as a dysregulation spectrum syndrome (DSS). DSS shares features with associated conditions such as spastic colitis and tension headache syndrome, in which a biologic and physiologic response to pain influences the psychological well-being of the patient. Theories of the 1970s that fibromyalgia was a somatization syndrome and others of the 1980s that it was a primary psychiatric disorder (affective spectrum disorder) have been shown to be invalid by advances in pain and neurotransmitter research. In addition, fibromyalgia patients do not have more psychotic, obsessive, hysterical, or hypochondriacal tendencies than one would find in the general population.

Part VI
IMPROVING YOUR QUALITY OF LIFE

Based on our experience, fewer than half of the 6 million Americans with fibromyalgia are taking prescription medication for complaints related to the syndrome. How do they get by? Whether or not formally diagnosed with fibromyalgia, these individuals (as well as those who take medication) instinctively make changes in their lifestyle. However, the quest for an improved quality of life is paved with uncertainties and unproven approaches. The next three chapters review how the symptoms and signs of fibromyalgia are influenced by daily activities and explore how approaches to diet, exercise, and personal interactions allow fibromyalgia patients to live a productive and fulfilling life.

18

Influences of Lifestyle and Environment on Fibromyalgia

A man cannot be comfortable without his own approval.
                Mark Twain (1835–1910), *What Is Man?* (1906)

Although there is no cure for fibromyalgia, patients can initiate numerous changes and make adjustments that improve their sense of well-being. Simply stated, there are things patients can do without spending money or seeing a health care provider. Demonstrating a certain amount of control over the syndrome also improves self-esteem and instills a sense of self-worth.

This chapter describes how modifications in diet, sleep habits, and lifestyle can ameliorate fibromyalgia. It also advises patients how best to deal with the weather, fatigue, pain, and their home environment so that they will hurt less and become more productive.

VITAMINS AND FOOD FOR THOUGHT: IS THERE A FIBROMYALGIA DIET?

What some call health, if purchased by perpetual anxiety
about diet, isn't much better than tedious disease.
        George Dennison Prentice (1802–1870), *Prenticeana*, 1860

Even though certain general dietary principles allow fibromyalgia patients to feel better, there is no "fibromyalgia diet." No specific food regimens or supplements have ever been shown in any published, controlled study to be helpful for fibromyalgia despite the observation that "arthritis diet" books are a multi-million-dollar-a-year industry.

How can we explain this discrepancy? First, people feel better when they eat healthy foods. Most "arthritis diet" books urge patients to eat three well-balanced meals a day and caution against overeating. Many recommend having the main meal at midday; heavy, late-evening dinners don't give the body enough time to burn off calories and are associated with bedtime esophageal spasm or heartburn. Similarly, consuming alcohol, nicotine, or caffeine (in the form of coffee, tea, or even chocolate) at a late dinner can make it harder to get a good night's sleep. In turn, poor sleep can increase musculoskeletal pain. An acceptable healthy balance of proteins, carbohydrates, and fats can also increase energy and fight fatigue.

What about vitamins? As people always on the go, Americans tend to settle for the convenience of quick-to-prepare, easy-to-consume refined, processed foods that are relatively deficient in vitamins and minerals. Multivitamin and mineral supplements can be useful additions for those who don't have time or are unable to prepare well-balanced meals. Many specialized formulas with heavily promoted "herbs and spices" are available from acquaintances, distributors, and health food stores; none of these have been shown to be superior to Wal-Mart, Rite-Aid, or Osco preparations available at a fraction of the cost. Most vitamins, herbs, minerals, and supplements added to multivitamins are harmless, but some are occasionally associated with allergic reactions (see Chapter 23).

Food sensitivity plays a role in less than 10 percent of our fibromyalgia patients. Within this group, different foods affect people differently. For example, some fibromyalgia patients feel better when they eat fish, while others hurt more. Some practitioners believe that carbohydrates increase serotonin levels, essential fatty acids diminish fatigue, and proteins improve mental alertness. Others place patients on a hypoglycemic/yeast elimination diet consisting of small, frequent meals, along with carbohydrate and wheat product restrictions. A few patients have had success with the Dong arthritis diet, a Duke University elimination diet that recognizes individual food sensitivity differences and provides a means for investigating what one can or cannot tolerate. We neither endorse nor refute any diet or food regimen for fibromyalgia, since none have been studied in a scientifically acceptable fashion. Thus, we have no admonitions for fibromyalgia patients regarding specific food groups.

BONING UP: DOES FIBROMYALGIA INTERACT WITH OSTEOPOROSIS?

As we age, our bones lose calcium. The loss of calcium leads to thinning of our bony architecture and affects its structural integrity. When bone mineralization decreases to a specified level, the consequences may lead to fracture. In the United States, 25 million Americans have *osteoporosis* (very thin bones), which is associated with 1.3 million fractures annually. Twenty percent of these fractures rob patients of the ability to live independently for varying periods of time, which results in pain management problems and loss of self-esteem.

The overwhelming majority of patients with osteoporosis are females, most of whom are menopausal. Although fibromyalgia does not cause or accelerate osteoporosis, it indirectly influences the disorder. For instance, exercise and other forms of physical activity help prevent calcium loss from the bone, while

Table 10. *Calcium supplementation.*

---

1. Foods with high calcium content (the average U.S. diet contains 600 mg a day)

Milk, 8 oz, 300 mg	Hard cheese, 1 oz, 200 mg
Ice cream, 1 cup, 176 mg	Oysters, 1/2 cup, raw, 113 mg
Broccoli, 1 cup, 136 mg	Sardines, canned, 3 oz, 372 mg
One large orange, 78 mg	Spinach, 1/2 cup raw, 111 mg
Yogurt, 8 oz, 400 mg	

2. Oral calcium supplements including examples of calcium products. Never take in over 600 mg at a time. The body does not absorb more. Reserve some calcium for bedtime.

    Calcium carbonate: OsCal, Tums, Titrilac, Maalox, Mylanta

    Calcium citrate: Citrical, Caltrate

    Calcium gluconate: Calcet

    Calcium lactate: store brands

3. Vitamin D improves the absorption of calcium by the gastrointestinal tract. The easiest way to derive enough vitamin D is by taking two multivitamin tablets a day.

---

smoking, poor nutrition, steroids, immobilization, and inactivity promote it. If fibromyalgia patients carry out the physical measures reviewed in Chapter 19, their risk of developing osteoporosis diminishes. From a dietary standpoint, it appears prudent to increase calcium in the diet or to supplement meals with at least 1.0 to 1.5 grams of calcium a day. Table 10 lists several ways this can be accomplished.

Bone mineralization can be assessed and quantitated by a variety of imaging studies, especially dual-energy X-ray absorptiometry (DEXA) scanning. Once osteoporosis is diagnosed or individuals at risk are identified, female hormones, a calcium hormone known as *calcitonin*, or drugs that prevent calcium loss from bones (known as *bisphosphonates*) may be prescribed.

ARE THERE MORE REASONS WHY SMOKING IS BAD?

Don't smoke. Its not only bad for obvious reasons, it also aggravates fibromyalgia. Nicotine is a stimulant, which can make it harder to sleep at night. Cigarettes induce hyperreactivity in airways in the lung, cause wheezing, and decrease stamina. Over time, smoking accelerates atherosclerosis, or hardening of the arteries, which diminishes the amount of oxygen delivered to muscles; this, in turn, can cause pain. Nicotine withdrawal has been associated with muscle spasms. Finally, vascular constriction or spasm caused by abnormal functioning of the ANS (see Chapter 7), observed in 30–40 percent of fibromyalgia patients, is worsened by smoking and leads to increased numbness, burning, and tingling.

In other words, there are absolutely no healthy reasons to smoke!

CAN FIBROMYALGIA BE BLAMED ON THE WEATHER?

Sunshine is delicious, rain is refreshing, wind braces us, snow is exhilarating; there is no such thing as bad weather, only different kinds of weather.

John Ruskin (1819–1900)

There is no question about it, nearly all patients feel that climate influences their fibromyalgia. In a recent survey, 66 percent of fibromyalgia patients related that they were affected by weather changes: 78 percent preferred warm weather, 79 percent believed that cold weather made them feel worse, and 60 percent did not like humidity. A variety of studies have suggested that musculoskeletal stiffness, achiness, and pain are aggravated by *changes* in barometric pressure. Fibromyalgia symptoms can be aggravated when the weather shifts from hot to cold or from wet to dry. A consistent climate is associated with fewer musculoskeletal symptoms. For instance, Hawaii theoretically has the perfect climate for fibromyalgia patients since it is usually within 4 degrees of 83°F and humid year round. However, before contacting a realtor, it's important to realize that this does not allow for changes in barometric pressure from walking into and out of air-conditioned buildings all day. What's the best way to deal with changes in climate? Don't panic or get upset if it takes a few days to acclimatize when traveling or if the weather changes.

Fibromyalgia patients living in northern climates are especially susceptible to a condition known as *seasonal affective disorder*. Light deprivation during the winter predisposes one to depression and fatigue. This can lead to decreased energy, productivity, motivation, libido, patience, and the ability to focus one's thoughts. Bright lights or a midwinter trip to Southern California, Arizona, or Florida can help break this form of emotional paralysis.

BUT I'M SO TIRED!

The feeling of sleepiness when you are not in bed and can't get there, is the meanest feeling in the world.

Edgar Watson Howe (1853–1937),
Country Town Sayings, 1911

Fatigue is a significant complaint in 75–80 percent of fibromyalgia patients. It can destroy relationships, lower self-esteem, and cause other people to accuse one of "making it up" since fibromyalgia patients generally look healthy. There are many things that can be done before considering medication. Once other medical problems that cause fatigue are ruled out, there are better ways to manage daily activities.

First, is the patient taking prescription medications (especially muscle relaxants) during the day that make them tired? Can alcohol or illicit drug use be a factor? The fibromyalgia patient should avoid daytime napping, after the early afternoon; otherwise it's harder to sleep at night. Many patients have overextended lives and, before becoming ill, were intensely active and overinvolved. Perfectionistic (but not obsessive) tendencies also can lead to fatigue since these individuals push to accomplish more than they are really able to do. It's important to establish realistic goals.

Here are a few tips on how to overcome fatigue. Most important, learn the concept of pacing. Be busy for a couple of hours in the morning and then take a 15- to 20-minute break. Engage in activities for another 2 hours and eat a leisurely lunch. Alternating periods of activity with rest times allow most fibromyalgia patients to be as productive as healthy people. Don't stay in bed all day trying to conserve energy. This can lead to depression, premature osteoporosis, atrophy of the muscles, flexion contractures, and *increased* pain over time because poor conditioning prevents muscles from getting enough oxygen.

If fatigue is an overwhelming problem, adopt a strategy to deal with it. First, get a good night's sleep and embark on a conditioning program. Plan ahead and try to accomplish only what is really important. Learn to have certain responsibilities handled by others and limit commitments. Within the confines of the pacing concept, learn to manage time, use energy wisely, and perform tasks requiring the greatest amount of focusing and energy at the time of day when functioning best. Many fibromyalgia patients have a midday "window" of feeling better—for example, from 10 A.M. to 2 P.M. Sometimes medications are given to decrease fatigue; these are reviewed in Chapter 22. Remember, there are many things that alleviate fatigue short of taking medicine.

I DON'T SLEEP WELL!

That we are not much sicker and much madder than we are is
due exclusively to that most blessed and blessing of all
natural graces, sleep.

Aldous Huxley (1894–1963),
Variations on a Philosopher, 1950

A good night's sleep is critical to overcoming fibromyalgia. Sleep heals our muscles and decreases daytime fatigue. Over 75 percent of fibromyalgia patients report significant sleep problems. The presentations of sleep complaints and a discussion of the biology of sleep in fibromyalgia were reviewed in Chapters 6 and 10.

Before considering a prescription sleep aid, there are many things that can be done to improve the sleep environment. First, take a look at the bedroom. Is the bed comfortable, the mattress firm, and the pillows suitable? A cervical pillow (our favorite is the Wal-Pil-O) reduces neck strain because it is shaped to support the neck. The room should be quiet and comfortable in temperature with a climate control system that keeps it neither too hot nor too cold. Don't let pets into the bedroom. Don't exercise vigorously after dinner. And allow the room to become dark before going to bed.

Start preparing for a good night's sleep early in the day. Don't nap after early afternoon. Don't drink a lot of fluids or take diuretics in the evening. Avoid caffeine, tobacco, alcohol, or a spicy or large meal too close to bedtime. On the other hand, don't starve, since hunger can also interfere with sleep. Use the hour before light's out to prepare for sleep. Think pleasing thoughts and practice slow, deep breathing. Soft music or relaxation tapes promote a restful mindset. Soak in a hot tub or take a hot shower and mentally close the day. Try not to read or listen to anything disturbing.

When the lights are turned out, one should fall asleep in 15–20 minutes. Falling asleep in less than 5 minutes suggests a state of sleep deprivation; on the other hand, if 30 minutes have elapsed, get up, since it's not time to sleep. With fibromyalgia, pain can make it difficult to fall or stay asleep, and patients need all the help they can muster. It may be more comfortable to lie on the back or side, or place a pillow under the knees to ease pressure on the lower back. If it's cold, consider using an electric blanket.

Once asleep, try to sleep enough to feel refreshed in the morning. Make sure bed partners do not snore to the point of interfering with needed rest. Don't keep the television or radio on. If you awaken at 3 A.M. and cannot sleep, get up and putter. The problem should take care of itself within a few nights.

These routines are inexpensive and easy to carry out. Many fibromyalgia patients can overcome sleep problems without medication if they focus attention on their sleep environment.

DOCTOR, I'M IN PAIN!

An hour of pain is as long as a day of pleasure.

English proverb

Pain is a natural sensation that is an unavoidable feature of fibromyalgia. Don't let it be controlling—learn to control it. In pain amplification syndromes such as fibromyalgia, distractions make us less aware of discomfort. Whether we are listening to music, driving a car, watching a movie, or performing work activities, pain perception is lessened when we don't concentrate on it. Biofeedback, meditation, and other techniques reviewed in Chapter 19 help send healing messages to painful areas. Fibromyalgia pain is never caused by and does not lead to crippling deformities. It's impossible to hurt yourself while "walking through the pain" by sublimating the sensation.

MAKING A HOUSE A HOME

Fibromyalgia may try to control the patient, but one way of fighting back is to create a home environment that minimizes the opportunity of producing discomfort. A little thought and organization can greatly improve the way one feels. In turn, this decreases pain without sapping precious energy reserves.

How can this be accomplished? Consolidate and simplify household chores — cook for two meals at once, take breaks, and perform only simple tasks when energy levels are low. Arrange activities to decrease the times needed to walk up and down stairs. Avoid putting things that get a lot of use in high cupboards. Use felt marker pens, which put less stress on the hands, and don't write for long periods of time. Of all the regular household activities, vacuuming is the worst. A vacuum cleaner's use aggravates back, shoulder, and arm discomfort and produces pain more often than any other appliance. Break up the activity. For starters, buy a lightweight vacuum cleaner and don't try to vacuum the whole house at once. When washing dishes, distribute body weight with one foot on a stepstool and try not to lean too far forward. Similarly, put one foot on a foot stool while ironing to reduce back strain. When washing windows, dusting, or scrubbing, find devices with longer, larger handles. If necessary, have somebody help carry in the groceries. Make your house more user friendly. If appropriate, change front door handles to levers, raise electrical outlets and phone jacks to a higher level, buy nonskid rugs, and use pull-out drawers or Lazy Susans.

Time and energy are too precious to squander—and this is one area where fibromyalgia patients have a lot of control.

AUTOMOBILES AND TRAVELING

It's important to get out and around, and most fibromyalgia patients travel in a car. Body mechanics in an automobile can make things better or worse. Bucket seats are more comfortable than bench seats. Make sure that the seat is adjustable and has armrests. The ideal vehicle for fibromyalgia patients should have an adequate headrest at the middle of the head for support, a climate control system, and automatic transmission. Mirrors should be plentiful, well placed, and easy to adjust. Don't recline, slouch, or sit too close to the steering column. For those with low back problems, buying a lumbar cushion or Sacro-Ease-like accessory may be useful.

While on vacation, take plenty of breaks from driving or sightseeing, find a flexible travel partner, and get a good night's sleep. Some fibromyalgia patients

bring their own neck collars or pillows with them. Don't be shy about using special luggage racks, carts, or wheels. Don't let isolation creep into your life—go
out, travel and enjoy!

HOW DO INFECTIONS INFLUENCE FIBROMYALGIA?

Most fibromyalgia patients have a normal immune system and don't get colds or
other infections more frequently than other people. However, infections can
aggravate fibromyalgia symptoms, and patients often take longer to recover. For
example, when fibromyalgia patients develop bronchitis, persistent coughing frequently intensifies myofascial pain in the upper back. Fevers decrease stamina to
a greater extent than in a healthy person. Viruses can lead to temporary relapses
of fatigue syndromes. It's important to cope with these frustrations in a productive way. Some fibromyalgia patients need to pace themselves and take it a bit
more slowly than usual for a little longer.

SUMMING UP

Certain aspects of life can be easily controlled. Fibromyalgia's impact can be
reduced by eating a healthy, well-balanced diet with appropriate vitamin and mineral supplements when needed, not smoking, minimizing the effects of changes
in barometric pressure, pacing, managing time, getting a good night's sleep, and
creating a home and travel environment that decreases activities known to produce fatigue, pain, and strain. The measures reviewed in this chapter are inexpensive, practical, and don't require visits to health care professionals.

19

The Influence of Exercise and Rehabilitation on the Mind and Body

We are under-exercised as a nation. We look instead of play.
We ride instead of walk. Our existence deprives us of the
minimum of physical activity essential for healthy living.
John F. Kennedy (1917–1963)

Let's continue on the self-help road to improving fibromyalgia symptoms. Suppose we are eating healthy, well-balanced meals, are no longer smoking, have learned to pace ourselves, cope with changes in the weather, are sleeping well, and have reconfigured the house. At this point, how can the body be trained to reduce pain, stiffness, and fatigue? This chapter will explore how physical, mental, and complementary modalities allow fibromyalgia patients to feel better about their bodies and minds.

PRINCIPLES OF FIBROMYALGIA REHABILITATION

Therapeutic regimens that help the body and mind, whether physical therapy, yoga, acupuncture, or chiropractic methods, are all based on similar tenets of body mechanics:

1. Fibromyalgia patients will never improve unless they have good posture. Bad posture aggravates musculoskeletal pain and creates tight, stiff, sore muscles. Therefore, stretch, change positions, and have a good workstation that does not require too much leaning or reaching.
2. The way we get around is a demonstration of body mechanics. The fundamental principles of good body mechanics in fibromyalgia include using a broad base of support by distributing loads to stronger joints with a greater surface area, keeping things close to the body to provide leverage, minimizing reaching, and not putting too much pressure on the lower back (demonstrated in Fig. 20). Also, don't stay in the same position for a prolonged period of time.

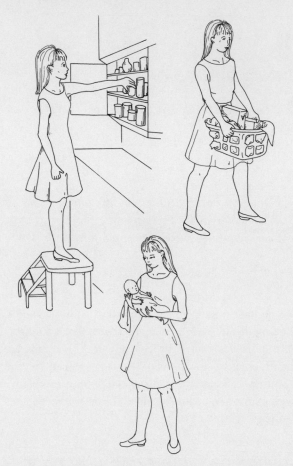

Fig. 20 *The basic principles of proper body mechanics that enhance well-being in fibromyalgia.*

3. Exercise is necessary. It improves our sense of well-being, strengthens muscles and bones, allows restful sleep, relieves stress, releases serotonin and endorphins, which decreases pain, and burns calories.
4. Don't be shy about using supports. Whether it be an armrest, special chair, brace, wall, railing, pillow, furniture, slings, pockets, or even another person's body, supports allow fibromyalgia patients to decrease the amount of weight or stress that would otherwise be applied to the body, producing discomfort or pain.
5. All activities should be conducive to relaxation and stress reduction, whether they be deep breathing, meditation, biofeedback, or guided imagery.

There is a surprisingly large number of ways these activities can be carried out. They are discussed in the next few sections.

PHYSICAL MODALITIES

The traditional methods for strengthening muscles, improving body mechanics and posture, and preventing damage are through exercise, physical therapy, and occupational therapy.

WHY DOES EXERCISING MAKE ME HURT MORE?

Many patients with fibromyalgia were physically quite vigorous before they developed the syndrome. A common complaint is that when they tried to resume their activities, exercise only increased their exhaustion and pain. A recent study showed that 83 percent of fibromyalgia patients do not exercise regularly and 80 percent are not considered physically fit. Some of the more common aggravating activities include heavy lifting or pulling. The CDC has even included "postexertion malaise" as a criterion for defining chronic fatigue syndrome. How can this paradox be explained?

As reviewed in Chapters 4–7, pain can result when muscles don't get enough oxygen. A consequence of changes in the ANS's signals is that this lack of oxygen and inefficient utilization of oxygen is further compounded by excessive constriction of blood vessels. In other words, when a fibromyalgia patient tries to exercise, a vicious cycle is unleashed. When blood vessels don't allow enough oxygen to be delivered to muscle tissue, even mild exercise produces microtrauma, or "angina," in muscles and pain. Further, microtrauma to the muscles can't be repaired at night since not enough growth hormone is released when we sleep poorly. In turn, these factors lead patients to avoid exercise in order to minimize discomfort. Over time, muscle atrophy, or wasting, and osteoporosis, or thinning of the bones, develop. This limits the patient's reserves and produces deconditioning so that even mild exertion results in profound fatigue.

What is the best kind of exercise for fibromyalgia?

How can fibromyalgia patients overcome the vicious cycle of exercise-pain-fatigue-exercise-pain-fatigue? First, motivation to undertake a gradual, progressive course of increasing activity and exercise is important. Try walking as the initial activity. Walk for 5 minutes twice a day, increasing to 45 minutes. Take breaks or sit on a bench if this makes you feel fatigued or winded. Walking is the first step toward a general conditioning and toning program. Over time, it relieves muscle and vascular spasm and allows more oxygen to reach the tissues. If the weather is bad, walk in an indoor mall. Walking with a friend can take the mind off what's going on, and time passes more easily.

Gradually, other general conditioning programs such as swimming and bicycling can be added to the regimen. Swimming for 30 to 60 minutes three times a week is an excellent way to strengthen muscles and condition the body. The buoyancy of water moves joints through their full range of motion and strengthens muscles with less stress, as you move in ways that are difficult outside of water. Swimmers bear only 10% of their body weight. While swimming, chest expansion allows for deeper breathing and more oxygen being taken in. Bicycling is an excellent activity that promotes general conditioning. Before buying a bicycle (stationary or otherwise), try it out and make sure the seat, handlebars, and amount of pedal resistance are comfortable.

Exercises are divided into several categories. In their simplest form, *isometric* exercises are useful in fibromyalgia. These routines allow patients to build muscle strength without moving, permitting a muscle to stretch until tension is felt. For example, the strap muscles in the neck can be strengthened by a cervical isometric program. If a patient pushes the forehead with moderate force against the hand placed against it and holds it for 6 seconds, the sustained muscle contraction (if repeated two times, twice a day along with other maneuvers as shown in Fig. 21) will strengthen the neck. This, in turn, protects patients against maneuvers, lurches, or sprains that increase upper back and lower neck strain. Along with isometric exercises, physical therapists frequently add *stretching* exercises to the regimen. Stretching does not allow jerking or bouncing around, decreases

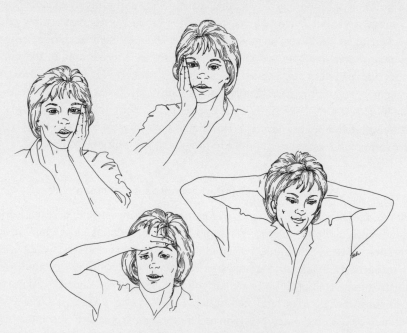

Fig. 21 *An example of strength-building isometric exercises. Performing these four cervical isometric maneuvers as sustained contractions for 6 seconds, twice a day, morning and evening, strengthens the sternocleidomastoid muscles and makes the neck less vulnerable to pain after injury or trauma.*

muscle tightness, prevents spasm and is performed together with deep-breathing exercises. Fibromyalgia patients often have shallow, jerky breathing patterns; slow, deep, rhythmic breathing promotes energy and allows relaxation.

Over time, patients work their way up to *isotonic* exercises that start with low-impact aerobics, where at least one foot is on the floor and there is no jumping. In their most helpful form, after a warmup period these activities allow enough arm and body movement to increase the heart rate without producing a jarring sensation that often makes fibromyalgia worse. We encourage fibromyalgia patients not to place too much tension on tender areas and have found that pain is accentuated by weight lifting, rowing, jogging or playing tennis, golf, or bowling early in the course of rehabilitation. Isotonic exercises are not for everybody and should be built up slowly. Make sure that a physician approves of the amount of exertion involved in an exercise program from a cardiovascular standpoint.

How can a physical therapist help fibromyalgia?

Physical therapists are health care professionals who usually have had 4–6 years of formal education after high school. They help patients achieve physical conditioning by using several modalities, especially the sorts of exercises reviewed above. Some additional modalities are the following:

1. *Massage* allows deep muscles to relax, loosens tight muscles, relieves pain and spasm, improves circulation, and decreases stress. Massages should be gentle so as not to aggravate fibromyalgia symptoms. The Alexander technique emphasizes posture and movement along with massage, and the Feldenkreis method incorporates massage with body-mind communication enhancements.

2. *Spray and stretch* is a technique by which a cool spray (ethyl chloride or fluori-methane) is applied to a painful area, numbing the nerves locally, and is followed by gentle stretching of the muscle underneath it, promoting relaxation.

3. *Heat* relaxes muscles and can be applied with the use of blankets, showers, waterbeds, hot tubs, lamps, microwave gelpacks, heating pads, or a hydroculator. Moist heat is usually more effective than dry heat. Therapists frequently use ultrasound to deliver deep heat to painful areas in a relaxing, rhythmic motion. These sound waves go to the muscles, tendons, and soft tissues. A variant of this technique is iontophoresis, in which medication such as xylocaine or a local steroid can be administered to painful areas. Temperatures above 90° F (such as in a jacuzzi or hot tub) should not be applied to any area of the body for longer than 15 minutes since the treatment can produce lightheadedness, dizziness, low blood pressure, or excessive fatigue.

4. *Ice* or cold packs treat injuries or strains less than 36 hours old by decreasing swelling. Approximately 15 percent of our fibromyalgia patients prefer cold to heat and benefit from ice massages. Icing an area for 10–15 minutes before vigorous activity (e.g., the shoulder before playing tennis or the shins prior to jogging) minimizes postexertional muscle pain in patients who are deconditioned.

5. *Electrical stimulation* delivers electrical impulses to nerves that, in turn, block painful messages. A form of electronic acupuncture, this can be accomplished by a TENS unit, acuscope, neuroprobe, or muscle exerciser.

6. Although chiropractors and osteopaths are known for their *manipulation* techniques, physical therapists also use traction, manipulation, and myofascial release.

7. *Posture and gait training* involves watching how patients walk and "carry" themselves. After evaluating a patient's body mechanics, the therapist may recommend strengthening and range-of-motion exercises, or assistive devices such as splints, collars, or braces.

8. The choice of *footwear* used while exercising or for everyday use is important. For the latter, the least expensive and most comfortable daily shoe is a sneaker a half size too big. For exercise, there should be no pressure on the sides or toe tips, heel counters should hold the heel firmly, and the shoe should be comfortable. Shoes with widened toe areas or Velcro straps rather than laces may be desirable.

9. Physical therapists often work with occupational therapists or counselors to assist patients with *relaxation techniques*. These include biofeedback, deep-breathing exercises, guided imagery, and meditation.

If you are getting physical therapy at a large institution, try to see the same therapist each time. Camaraderie and close working relationships are associated with better outcomes.

What is an occupational therapist?

The term *occupational therapist* is a very misleading. Vocational rehabilitation counselors, not occupational therapists, advise patients about what employment is best for them and arrange for appropriate coursework and training. Occupational therapists practice a discipline known as *ergonomics* in designing work tasks to fit the capabilities of the human body (see Chapter 24). They perform an ADL, or Activities of Daily Living Evaluation. Occupational therapists consider such questions as: How much energy do people waste performing various chores such as housework? Is there a better way to get into and out of a car, on and off a toilet seat, or into and out of a bathtub? Occupational therapists apply principles of energy conservation and joint protection in their evaluations. Many large companies have therapists on site to evaluate workstations, office furniture, computer screen levels, and distances. Is the office environment smoke free, aesthetically pleasing, and user friendly? (See Chapter 24.) Is there adaptive equipment such as a longer or thicker handle that decreases reaching, bending, or lifting? Is splinting or bracing useful? Occupational therapists are experts when it comes to using or designing special wheels, levers, lightweight objects, enlarged handles, or specialized convenience tools. In our opinion, these underutilized professionals are unsung heroes responsible for a portion of the increased corporate productivity that the United States has enjoyed over the last 20 years.

When is a physical or occupational therapy evaluation useful?

In our experience, patients with mild fibromyalgia infrequently need a formal rehabilitation program. Many physical therapists have little training concerning the needs of fibromyalgia patients and should consider taking a course the Arthritis Foundation offers to be up-to-date. Unfortunately, only one-third of our patients tell us that physical therapy was very useful, one-third report that they felt fine for a few hours afterward before returning to their baseline condition, and one-third say that they felt worse because the program was too aggressive or hard on the soft tissues. In the hands of highly proficient physical and occupational therapists, chronically ill patients or those refractory to treatment can have dramatic responses to a well-designed, well-thought-out rehabilitation program. An outstanding example with a high published success rate is the program devised by Drs. Sharon Clark and Robert Bennett at the University of Oregon Heath Sciences Center in Portland.

We usually prescribe physical and occupational therapy in tandem with medication to our patients who perform moderate to severe activity. The ideal program consists of 12–16 45-minute sessions over 3–4 months, after which patients can exercise independently and do their own rehabilitation. Most insurance carriers will pay for 10–20 physical therapy sessions a year if the need is well documented. About 10 percent of our fibromyalgia patients, especially those with reflex sympathetic dystrophy, benefit from 1 or 2 years of physical therapy.

MENTAL MODALITIES

Anybody who is 25 or 30 years old has physical scars from all sorts
of things, from tuberculosis to polio. It's all the same with the mind.
Ralph Kaufman, 20th-century health practitioner

Mental health professionals have become increasingly interested in using their expertise and resources to help fibromyalgia patients. *Psychiatrists* are medical doctors and can prescribe medication. *Psychologists* have a master's degree or a doctorate, are not physicians, and cannot prescribe medication. *Medical or psychiatric social workers* frequently work with psychologists and psychiatrists and provide counseling services. Some *nurse practitioners* have specialized psychiatric training. Members of the *clergy* frequently fulfill a healing role in advising and assisting fibromyalgia patients. Most have some training, and many have degrees in psychology, counseling, or social work. Traditionally, these health professionals use a variety of techniques to decrease stress, enhance coping skills, diminish fatigue, build self-esteem, and improve interpersonal interactions. Patients must feel comfortable with their therapists, and there should be a minimum of distraction during therapy sessions.

Classical psychotherapy

We refer 10–20 percent of our fibromyalgia patients to psychotherapists. Fibromyalgia patients who are the best candidates for classical psychotherapy are in touch with reality and capable of having stable relationships with people, looking at themselves realistically, and being introspective. They should be willing to accept personal responsibility, have no secondary gain from their symptoms, and be interested in learning how to deal with anxiety, anger, or frustration without "acting out." The goals of therapy sessions are to verbalize concerns, confront inappropriate behavior patterns, clarify or understand these patterns based on past experiences, and work through problems. Patients should be able to identify their fears and destructive thinking patterns. They should try not to blame or make broad judgments. The treating professional and patient must form a therapeutic alliance enabling patients to develop a constructive means for dealing with problems that are prolonging stress, fatigue, or pain.

Cognitive therapy: An newer approach to "brain fatigue"

Cognitive therapy is a useful approach for patients with fibromyalgia who have difficulty learning, retaining, processing, recalling, finding words, focusing, concentrating, planning, or organizing. Cognitive dysfunction or impairment is usually intermittent and probably reflects spasm of blood vessels supplying oxygen to the brain as part of a dysfunctioning ANS (see Chapter 7). Most patients who report cognitive symptoms note that they are intermittent and of short duration. However, up to 10 percent of our patients have had to alter their lifestyle to accommodate cognitive symptoms.

Cognitive therapists usually are psychologists, occupational therapists, or speech therapists. They urge their clients to use memory aids such as placing project lists and Post-its around the house, decrease distractions, form mental pictures to assist with associations, and not to get frustrated when trying to find words. Bad moods, depression, and anxiety can have a negative influence on memory. Therapists show patients how to use cues, designate one spot at home as the repository of all knowledge, and write things down so that they will not forget. Having regular daily routines, using timers or alarm clocks, and having a regular filing system also are useful. Be frank about the problem; covering up "brain fatigue" only makes things worse.

Stress reduction strategies and biofeedback

Relaxation decreases SNS activity, slows the heart rate, and improves oxygen delivery to the muscles and brain. In particular, fibromyalgia patients have a heightened awareness of their autonomic functions such as pulse, blood pressure, and muscle tone. One of the most popular relaxation techniques is *biofeedback*, which teaches patients to control their body responses in order to minimize anxiety, provide relaxation, and promote pain relief. Electrical monitors can record skin temperature, heart rate, brain waves, and electrical skin conductivity (which measures muscle tension and is termed *EMG biofeedback*). Although at first glance it may seem like hocus-pocus, study after study has shown that deep-breathing exercises, relaxation tapes, and visualizing pleasant environments (called *guided imagery*) promote endorphin release and decrease muscle tension, pain, and stress. *EEG biofeedback* blocks some types of brain waves (reviewed in the sleep section of Chapter 10) and reinforces others to improve cognitive, perceptual, and sleeping skills. Biofeedback can be administered by physicians, physical therapists, occupational therapists, or psychologists and is usually covered by insurance if the need for it is well documented.

Several controlled studies have shown that *cognitive behavioral therapy* improves fibromyalgia. These programs combine education, cognitive behavioral intervention, stress reduction techniques, support for family members and spouses, and strategies to improve physical fitness and flexibility. Biofeedback incorporates meditation, as do other techniques. For example, *yoga* combines deep breathing, meditation, and specific postures that integrate mental, physical, and spiritual energies to enhance well-being. *Transcendental meditation* enables patients to focus on a single thought or object to create an inner calm which banishes stress. *T'ai chi* adds passive movements to achieve this result. Also, never underestimate the power of *prayer* along with quiet contemplation.

COMPLEMENTARY MODALITIES
(ALTERNATIVE THERAPIES)

Formerly known as *alternative medicine*, complementary medicine approaches are defined as nontraditional therapeutic approaches practiced by physicians or health care professionals. In general, very few of these disciplines are taught in conventional medical schools. Why should we bother talking about complementary therapies? Simply because mainstream practitioners do not have all the answers, and some patients improve with these interventions. Why else would the U.S. public spend $14 billion a year on complementary therapies, mostly out of their own pockets? While some complementary modalities such as chiropractic are widely used and well established, others clearly have no place in managing fibromyalgia. This section will review some of these modalities. Homeopathy is covered in Chapter 23, and some complementary meditation techniques were reviewed in the previous section.

Does acupuncture work?

According to ancient Chinese tradition, yin and yang are complementary aspects of chi, an energizing life force energy. Chi flows in the body through meridians, or imaginary lines along which the principles of acupuncture are based. Fine-gauge, sterilized needles are inserted along these meridians to allow "energy paths" signaling the brain to heal pain. Used for over 2500 years, acupuncture ideally should stimulate endorphin release and diminish pain in fibromyalgia tender points. In our experience, acupuncture is safe and inexpensive. The use of electrical acupuncture (see the physical therapy section of this chapter) is not restricted to the traditional meridians in relieving tender point pain. Most rheumatologists find the results of traditional acupuncture to be modest at best in managing fibromyalgia.

How do osteopaths treat fibromyalgia?

The discipline of osteopathy was founded by Andrew Taylor Still (1828–1917), an American physician who served as a surgeon during the Civil War. Frustrated by illogical therapies employed by organized medicine at the time, Dr. Still hypothesized that an integrated and balanced musculoskeletal structure was optimal for physiological functioning. Further, the body's structural function depended upon psychological, emotional, familial, and societal influences. The 17 osteopathic medical schools in the United States train doctors almost the same way as medical schools that award an M.D. (medical doctor) degree as opposed to a D.O. (doctor of osteopathic) degree. Most of the 50,000 osteopaths practice in a primary care, family practice, or internal medicine setting. However, their training also includes instruction in physical modalities such as myofascial release, cranial manipulation, and high-velocity, low-amplitude "thrusts," which benefit many of our fibromyalgia patients. Over the years, some of these techniques have found their way into general use by rehabilitation medicine physicians, physical therapists, and chiropractors.

How do chiropractors manage fibromyalgia?

In 1895, an Iowa healer named D. D. Palmer developed the theory that proper alignment of the spinal column allows unimpeded nerve flow to the soft tissues. This flow is necessary to achieve optimal health. If structural bones and body muscles are in proper alignment, the body should take over and heal itself. Unlike osteopaths, chiropractors do not practice internal medicine, perform surgery, or write prescriptions. In an effort to treat spinal *subluxations* (less than full dislocations), they use manual adjustments, manipulations, and "cracking" to force movements of body parts to increase range of motion and relax muscles. There are 45,000 chiropractors in the United States, and 10 percent of the population visits them at least occasionally. Over the years, chiropractors have incorporated principles of rehabilitation medicine, physical therapy, occupational therapy, and osteopathy into their practice. We have found that their interventions generally are modestly beneficial to our fibromyalgia patients. Patients who seek chiropractic therapy should coordinate the modalities employed with their primary care physician, rheumatologist, physiatrist, or orthopedist. The only controlled trial of chiropractic in fibromyalgia had negative results. There are many ways health care professionals can work together to improve their patients' health. Occasionally, some chiropractic approaches aggravate fibromyalgia-related pain. If this is the case, therapy should either be discontinued or discussed with the physician and chiropractor.

Investigational or questionable complementary approaches

Naturopathy is based on the belief that disease can be treated by a return to nature in regulating the diet, deep-breathing exercises, bathing, and the employment of various forces to eliminate poisonous products from the system. While there is nothing wrong with using the healing powers of nature, in our opinion laxatives, purges that induce vomiting, and colonics are of no benefit for fibromyalgia and are potentially dangerous. The *ayurveda* uses yoga and dietary modifications that present no problems, but also preaches that correct spiritual and physical balancing requires purification. These purifications include enemas, vomiting, and blood letting, which only aggravate fibromyalgia. *Reflexology* treats the ears, hands, and feet with manual stimulation as a way of treating the whole body. Based on the theory that specific areas of the ears, hands, and feet correspond to organs, glands, and nerves, reflexology makes no scientific sense but may help patients through a placebo effect in giving them time, attention, relaxation, and a sympathetic ear. As noted earlier in this chapter, many forms of *massage* clearly benefit patients. However, specific massage techniques such as rolfing and hellerwork are too vigorous for most fibromyalgia patients and frequently induce more pain. These techniques may be appropriate for patients without fibromyalgia. Finally, the belief that *magnetic fields* influence energy and blood flow has had a resurgence of popularity since the introduction of MRI imaging as a diagnostic procedure. Some advocates of the *polarity theory* believe that magnets can balance energy forces of the body and apply magnets to various areas of the body. None of our patients who have done this have had any response to this treatment, for which there is little scientific basis.

SUMMING UP

A minority of fibromyalgia patients require a formalized rehabilitation program. When prescribed, it generally consists of a gradual exercise program, as well as physical and occupational therapy. Some form of counseling may be part of this program. The principal goals of any rehabilitation process should include reducing stress, promoting greater stamina and endurance, improving clarity of thought, avoiding discomfort at work and at home, showing patients how to carry on an independent exercise program, lessening reliance on medication, and improving the ability to cope with pain.

20

How to Overcome Fibromyalgia

*All living souls welcome whatever they are ready to cope
with; all else they ignore, or pronounce to be monstrous and
wrong, or deny to be possible.*

George Santayana (1863–1952),
Dialogues in Limbo, 1925

When our patients are diagnosed with fibromyalgia, their initial reaction generally is "What?" At this point, we provide them with literature from fibromyalgia
support groups and the Arthritis Foundation and explain what this condition
means. Often we meet with family members to reinforce the educational process.
In mild cases, this creates a sense of relief. Some patients who have seen several
physicians and been given various diagnoses have differing reactions: "Are you
just trying to put me off?" "My last rheumatologist said the same thing, told me
he could do nothing for it, and sent me back to my family doctor." "Are you sure
it's not lupus or Lyme disease or cancer?"

Once our patients have accepted the diagnosis and read about the syndrome,
we examine their behavior patterns and try to find ways to help them deal with the
diagnosis in a constructive manner. This chapter reviews some of the emotional
reactions our patients display and problems they have to deal with, gives practical
advice on how to surmount obstacles, and describes community resources that
help patients overcome the syndrome.

THE PROBLEM: WHY COPING IS DIFFICULT

It's hard enough to get through the day when feeling unwell. In fibromyalgia, the
sense of being unwell is manifested by fatigue, pain, spasm, poor sleeping, lack
of stamina or endurance, and sometimes difficulty concentrating or focusing.
Fibromyalgia patients frequently react to these sensations with specific attitudes,
emotions, and other behavioral responses, including anxiety, anger, guilt, loss of
self-esteem, depression, and fear.

You look great! How could you be sick?

There are no physical markers of fibromyalgia that reveal the syndrome to others. Fibromyalgia patients have no deformities, don't have an X marked on their

forehead, look healthy, and seem able to be active. While this is good for the patient in one sense, friends, employers, and loved ones often have difficulty believing that they have so many complaints. Therefore, it's important to be open and frank with those who care. You need to have their trust to help them understand the limitations imposed by fibromyalgia. Patients do not need to be coddled or treated like invalids; they crave and need understanding and respect. Tell those who care that with a few modifications and a little time, you can still be as productive and as much fun to be with as before.

Anxiety

Anxiety is fear of one's self.
Wilhelm Stekel

Anxiety is present in up to 70 percent of patients with fibromyalgia at some point during the course of the syndrome. It can be manifested by shortness of breath, palpitations, dizziness, lightheadedness, sweaty palms, trembling, chest pains, nausea, hot flashes, and, in extreme cases, a sense of impending doom or panic. Anxiety, in turn, worsens fibromyalgia symptoms, which sometimes can be hard to differentiate from those of anxiety. Anxiety is distressing but, if confronted firmly, will pass. Examine the causes of anxiety, face them, and don't run away. Patients must learn to relax and master their minds and bodies. Practice deep breathing, try to create a comfortable environment, write, or listen to pleasant music. Find ways to get a sense of control, dissipate the tensions of the day, create a sense of well-being, and get a good night's sleep.

Loss of self-esteem

Be a friend to thyself, and others will be so too.
Thomas Fuller, M.D. (1654–1734),
Gnomologia, 1732

Fibromyalgia is a formidable syndrome that can lead to loss of self-esteem. Hurting and being tired all the time takes its toll. Some patients cannot meet educational or career goals, lose the ability to be self-supporting, cannot engage in community activities, or experience cognitive impairment and difficulty focusing. This may lead to unstable or failed relationships with family and friends, with consequent loss of self-esteem.

The first thing a fibromyalgia patient needs to be aware of is a self-esteem problem. How did this happen? What can be done about it? Several steps can improve self-esteem in a fibromyalgia patient. Achieving a sense of personal worth promotes self-confidence. Visualize being happy. Do things that are enjoyable or help others. Stop being negative. Develop affirmations: I am courageous; I have options; I am not a victim; I am learning to relax; I can solve it. Peer counseling is frequently helpful in this situation. Getting back one's self-esteem is one of the first steps toward overcoming fibromyalgia.

Anger

It's my rule never to lose my temper until it would be detrimental to keep it.

Sean O' Casey (1884–1964),
The Plough and the Stars, 1926

Patients who get upset because they are not feeling well aggravate their fibromyalgia by tightening their muscles, making relaxation impossible. There are several self-help steps to confronting anger. First, conduct a personal reality check. Is there anything actually wrong with the way things are going? Are your loved ones healthy and alive? How are things financially? Don't get upset over things beyond your control, such as traffic jams or long lines at the supermarket. Deal with life's stresses in nonconfrontational ways. When making phone calls that require being on hold for a while, watch television or listen to music while waiting. Don't run errands that might require standing in long lines if time is a problem. Don't blame people for causing your problems or illness. Anger can be energizing, but channel it positively. There are healthy ways to express bottled-up anger. Think of how to prevent getting angry and how to relieve anger when it builds. Keep a chart or diary to award accomplishments in dealing with problems. It will help create a sense of well-being.

Guilt and shame

Guilt, once harbored in the conscious breast, intimidates the brave, degrades the great.

Samuel Johnson (1709–1784)

Guilt has no place in fibromyalgia and makes the syndrome worse. Try to recognize its destructive effects. Regretting past behavior or thinking that you are bad are attitudes to be avoided. Don't berate yourself for things that fibromyalgia does not allow you to do. Overly perfectionistic tendencies can lead to guilt, as can unrealistic goal setting. Don't agonize over decisions that may have had unintended outcomes. We are all human, and we all make mistakes. Propose a rational response for dealing with guilt and looking ahead. Guilt is self-defeating. Develop a positive attitude to modify thoughts and behavior.

Depression

You handle depression in much the same way you handle a
tiger. . . . If depression is creeping up and must be faced,
learn something about the nature of the beast: you may
escape without a mauling.

R. W. Shepherd

In Chapter 17, we reviewed evidence that patients do not develop fibromyalgia because they are depressed, but that they can be depressed because
they do not feel well. This reactive depression manifests as loss of interest
and pleasure in life's daily activities. Classically defined as "helplessness and
hopelessness," depression leads to a feeling of worthlessness, loss of appetite
(or occasionally overeating), altered sleep patterns, loss of self-esteem, inability
to concentrate, guilt, complaints of fatigue, and loss of energy. Patients who
are depressed have lower pain thresholds, lose interest in personal care and
grooming, have trouble making decisions, and sometimes get into more acci-
dents or arguments. Depression affects the body, moods, relationships, and physical activities.

In order to overcome depression, fibromyalgia patients must first recognize
that it's a problem and express a desire to do something about it. Once an ounce
of motivation is kindled, some of the techniques discussed in Chapter 19 and
later on in this chapter can be used to fight off depression. Medications prescribed to manage depression are reviewed in the next two chapters.

Perfectionism

Striving to better, oft we mar what's well.
Shakespeare (1564–1606),
King Lear, Act 1, sc. 4, l. 369

Many of our fibromyalgia patients are overachievers. Prior to becoming ill, they
led very busy lives with personal, work, and societal commitments. A perfectionistic tendency is evident where every detail of each daily activity is comprehen-
sively thought out and analyzed. This needs to be differentiated from a psychiatric disorder known as obsessive-compulsive behavior, which is reviewed in
Chapter 17 and is not associated with fibromyalgia. When the symptoms of
fibromyalgia manifest themselves, fatigue makes it difficult to accomplish all the
patient is able to do, which in turn creates feelings of guilt and inadequacy when
the patient cannot perform. This leads to fears of failure and rejection and difficulty handling criticism. Overachievers need to adjust, think innovatively, learn
to budget their energy, and delegate responsibility. Don't get so bogged down in

detail that the overall picture is lost. Let initial frustrations evolve into relaxation. Life is too precious to waste on details beyond our control!

Fear and trauma

The only thing we have to fear is fear itself—nameless, unreasoning, unjustified terror which paralyzes needed efforts to convert retreat into advance.

> Franklin D. Roosevelt (1882–1945),
> *Inaugural Address*, 1933

A minority of patients with fibromyalgia had something terrible happen to them in the past, which makes it harder to overcome pain, poor sleeping patterns, and spasm. They may have been a victim of abuse, neglect, a natural disaster, war, poverty, or a crime. Don't let others convince these patients that a single factor such as a virus, a specific diet, or a genetic tendency is solely responsible for the illness. Counseling is absolutely critical. Patients need to verbalize their traumas and the fears that go with them. They need to confront the facts of the situation and work out a way to get the past behind them so that their lives can go forward. This may require relocating to a safer environment, ending abusive relationships, or altering work styles. Only at this point can fibromyalgia be effectively overcome.

SOLUTIONS: HOW TO IMPROVE COPING SKILLS

As we have demonstrated, anxiety, fear, guilt, depression, loss of self-esteem, and anger are common emotions found in fibromyalgia patients. How should patients deal with these emotions and learn to cope better? Adequate coping requires taking action. Fasten your seat belts. We are going to do just that!

Develop positive goals and attitudes

Holly was gorgeous and the envy of her friends. She always seemed in control and worked 18 hours a day building her communications consulting business. No detail was too small to be overlooked. But over several months, the fragile shell that nobody knew she had started to crack. After what seemed to be a mild flu, she began sleeping poorly and complaining of muscle spasms. Of course, Holly kept this to herself. However, when she started forgetting telephone numbers and a splitting headache nearly caused her to miss an important meeting, Holly consulted Dr. Gray. The workup showed that Holly had fibromyalgia. Her perfectionistic tendencies enabled Holly to block the problem she was having forming serious relationships. Holly was lonely, and her family was 2000 miles away.

Her immediate reaction was anger, which gave way to chronic anxiety. Although she reduced her workload, this only created a feeling of guilt. Dr. Gray referred her to a psychologist, who explained to Holly that her pain amplification was real and probably virally induced, but that unless she faced up to things in a positive, constructive manner, improvement would be much slower. Holly learned to manage her time and think positively. She learned how to relax and channel her frustration into energizing activities. Holly allowed herself time to go out on dates and rediscovered her sense of humor. She no longer takes fibromyalgia medication.

Patients should treat the diagnosis of fibromyalgia as a challenge to their resourcefulness. Like Holly, they should set realistic goals and be proactive. List all the problems, from easiest to hardest to resolve. Write down the remedies for each symptom, sign, and problem, one at a time. Follow the results. Reprioritize goals. Try not to do annoying, recurrent tasks. Don't be drawn into a no-win situation. Set limits and learn to say no. Avoid negative people. Instead of thinking that "It's hopeless and will never get better" or "This treatment will make me worse," try developing the attitude that things will get better and medication will help. Discuss medications with a doctor and inquire how they assist self-improvement. Decide if individual or group counseling is something that might expedite more positive feelings.

It's important to do positive things by challenging one's financial, personal, and intellectual resources. Cultivate spirituality. Develop new interests and hobbies. Seek positive news and information. Improve communication skills. If you are courteous and say "please" and "thank you," others will be helpful and pleasant in return. Give affection to others, and it will be returned. Don't worry about tomorrow; focus on what can be done today. Be open to receiving help and verbalizing thoughts; don't keep them suppressed. Patients who set attitude changes as goals really do start to feel better about themselves.

How to improve coping

Laurel always had low self-esteem. She worked installing turbines on an assembly line for a small, family-owned technology company. After several weeks, the pressure of carrying 50-pound boxes to the assembly area got to her. Laurel complained of pain in her back and shoulders and tingling in her hands. Over the next few months she found it increasingly difficult to sleep, and her abdomen became so distended that a friend asked her if she was pregnant. Laurel quit work after 5 months, but the pain did not go away. Dr. Lane noted that Laurel also reported headaches, palpitations, fatigue, low back discomfort, and stools filled with mucus. A diagnosis of fibromyalgia with irritable bowel syndrome was made. Her inability to hold the job made Laurel depressed and destroyed her self-confidence.

She seemed to be teary-eyed most of the time and was motivated to do nothing other than watch television and eat potato chips. Dr. Lane prescribed half a tablet of cyclobenzaprine (Flexeril) 2 hours before sleeping and Levsin for her bowel discomfort, and a week later added fluoxetane (Prozac) in the morning. Since Laurel had lost her health insurance and could not afford counseling, Dr. Lane referred her to a local fibromyalgia support group, and Laurel took the Arthritis Foundation's "Fibromyalgia Self-Help Course." The course showed Laurel how to develop self-confidence and a positive outlook. Several months later, Laurel got a clerking job through a friend she met at the course and has held it for the past year. Dr. Lane intends to taper her medications soon.

In order to cope with fibromyalgia, be flexible and learn to adapt to the illness. Life can be happy in spite of fibromyalgia. Learn to understand the concept of self-responsibility and accept it. Most patients work, despite feeling unwell, by accommodating the illness. Explain what fibromyalgia is to spouses, relatives, and friends. The importance of seeking help and avoiding isolation cannot be overemphasized.

Dealing with stress

Fern was getting it from all sides. Her mother had recently died, her son's business had gone bankrupt, and a flood caused severe damage to the home she had lived in for 30 years. Fern's stable fibromyalgia flared, and her lower back and neck pain was excruciating. Determined to overcome these obstacles, Fern took stock of herself. Her children were healthy, the house was insured, and she was happily married. She took alprazolam (Xanax) for 3 nights to alleviate the anxiety that had prevented her from sleeping. Fern rejoined her exercise class, which included deep-breathing exercises, stretching, and nonimpact aerobics. Every morning, she performed isometric exercises for 10 minutes. Whenever her husband noticed early signs of an inappropriate stress response, he made a point of warning her that she was getting anxious. Fern responded by practicing a biofeedback maneuver she had learned. She stopped volunteer work at an agency where her efforts were not appreciated and the work was too time-consuming. She made sure that there was time for herself during the day. Fern's fibromyalgia started to ease up.

In Chapters 3 and 6, we reviewed how stress or trauma can bring on fibromyalgia and reviewed the biochemical pathways by which this occurs. A recent survey suggested that 63 percent of fibromyalgia patients feel that stress is a major factor in influencing their symptoms, signs, and disease course.

How can stress be decreased? First, remember that lessening stress increases energy. In the beginning, learn to relax. Find a quiet environment and a comfortable position. Whether it's listening to soft music, practicing meditation, guided imagery, deep abdominal breathing, hypnosis, thinking of or inhaling pleasant aromas (*aromatherapy*), t'ai chi, prayer, or biofeedback, we support whatever works. Next, learn to say no and communicate your concerns. It may be necessary to accept limitations and modify job descriptions and workstations to limit physical and emotional stress. Budget time to allow for periods of relaxation. Learn to pace. Make a list of everything that is stressful and how these factors can be avoided or improved. Also, enjoy distractions. Have fun. Learn to laugh. Listen to comedy shows or tapes, read a good book, or take up gardening. Get a pet. Develop a hobby. Distractions make it easier to perform necessary or required activities that are less enjoyable. Finally, remember that stress can cause and aggravate fibromyalgia by releasing chemicals that aggravate or accelerate symptoms of pain and fatigue.

Develop a positive doctor-patient relationship

Never go to a doctor whose office plants have died.
Erma Bombeck (1927–1996)

Whether they are seeing a mental health therapist, physical therapist, chiropractor, or physician, patients must be able to communicate with their health care professional. Since only physicians can prescribe medication or hospitalize, their relationships with and feelings toward patients are extremely important. Here are a few tips on how to maximize the doctor-patient relationship.

Find a doctor who believes that fibromyalgia exists and is interested in helping these patients. Avoid unreasonable expectations. Does the doctor have a genuine interest in the patient as a person? Does the physician reinforce the patient's self-esteem, listen, or allow disagreements or questions? Does the patient feel comfortable asking questions or feel too rushed? Does the doctor talk in plain English? Most important, will the doctor be the patient's advocate? Can he or she write jury duty letters, allow handicap placards if needed, fill out disability forms, and defend the patient in a legal deposition?

In return for these considerations, be sensitive to the doctor's needs. Be organized and honest. If it's hard to explain a problem, write it down and restrict the note to one page. What makes the complaint better or worse? What's been tried in the past? Do not argue with the doctor. Be informative and reasonable. Don't expect an instant cure. Follow the suggested course of therapy to completion—a noncompliant patient cannot expect to improve fully. Doctor-patient relationships are important partnerships that can be quite fragile at times.

If a physician referral is needed, call the nearest medical school, county medical association, Arthritis Foundation, or fibromyalgia support group.

HOW TO MOBILIZE RESOURCES

There are many people who really care about a fibromyalgia patient's health and well-being. Whether it be a spouse, family member, friend, or someone in the community, there are many resources that can be called upon in the treatment process. In the following sections, we describe the kinds of help that support people and groups can provide.

Marriage, sexuality, and family

Pains do not hold a marriage together. It is threads, hundreds of tiny threads which sew people together through the years. . . . That's what makes a marriage last—more than passion or even sex.

Simone Signoret (1921–1985)

Marge had been married to Henry for 5 years when she sustained a whiplash injury in a motor vehicle accident. Though she did all the right things, her localized neck sprain evolved into full-blown fibromyalgia over several months. Marge complained of fatigue, aching, and irritable colon. She became sensitive to weather changes and had difficulty sleeping. Since she looked the same, Henry could not understand why Marge would not play golf with him on weekends or why she kept him up at night tossing and turning while trying to find a comfortable position. Henry's anger made things worse, and this affected their relationship. A classmate of Marge's sister at the university had fibromyalgia. The classmate's advice to the sister allowed Marge to confide her concerns to her parents and siblings. Marge rented a video on fibromyalgia from the Arthritis Foundation for Henry since he did not like to read. She took Henry to her next rheumatology visit, and Dr. March explained how Henry could be more understanding and supportive. Henry demonstrated greater insight, which indirectly helped Marge's fibromyalgia to improve.

Married or unmarried couples may wish to probe how their relationship interacts with fibromyalgia and vice versa. Make sure that the partner knows what fibromyalgia is and how he or she can help the patient enjoy life. Open communication decreases resentment and resolves potential conflict. Be on the lookout for potential problems. Does the partner resent or attempt to control the fibromyalgia patient? Does he or she buffer upsetting information before telling the patient? Does the mate derive satisfaction from caring for a fibromyalgia patient? Does the mate feel neglected or unable to help?

A good sexual relationship is a source of pleasure, self-esteem, and relaxation, which also decreases stress. Fibromyalgia should not interfere physiologically with lovemaking. The uncommon exceptions include autonomically mediated dry vaginal walls (easily treated with lubricants) and significant spasm of vaginal muscles, often with a history of sexual or physical abuse (see Chapter 13). Occasionally, fibromyalgia medications can influence libido. Don't be afraid to ask a doctor about the potential side effects of medications before taking them. Enhancing intimacy while reducing stress should be a goal.

Relatives and friends should be helpful resources. Some fibromyalgia patients react to the disease by decreasing their social contacts and isolating themselves. "I'm too tired to do anything" or "I hurt too much to be away for more than a few hours" are warning signs of a developing problem. When patients complain of difficulty keeping up with household chores or meeting responsibilities to their children, relationships may become precarious. The sleep disorder of fibromyalgia can also alter intimacy. Develop a positive plan to be an active family member, taking limitations into account. Keep all communication channels open with family members. They should be a patient's biggest cheerleaders!

Sometimes, family strife can worsen fibromyalgia. If this is the case, identify the sources of stress that interfere with rehabilitation. Focus on the problems, develop means for dealing with them positively, and seek counseling if needed.

Community resources and self-help groups

In addition to a doctor, health care professional, family, mate, and friends, there are community resources. For example, many Arthritis Foundation chapters conduct a "Fibromyalgia Self-Help Course." It educates patients about fibromyalgia and trains leaders, who in turn are able to lead rap groups or self-help sessions. They meet once a week for 2 to 3 hours over several weeks. Other fibromyalgia support organizations also have lists of patients and doctors in different areas of 0the country who are interested in the syndrome. Appendix 1 lists other agencies and organizations that assist fibromyalgia patients.

A self-help group usually consists of 5–20 members who meet on a regular basis (usually once a month) to share information and experiences. The group leader should allow time for questions and answers, give research and clinical updates, and permit presentations by health care professionals. The leader should be strong yet empathetic, not allow one person to dominate the sessions, and set a positive, constructive tone. Members develop friendships that often provide additional support systems.

Finally, we need to address the Internet. Fibromyalgia patients surfing the Internet will find three basic sources of information: legitimate research and summaries of clinical papers put together by fibromyalgia support organizations or medical society Web sites; entrepreneurs trying to sell dietary or medically unproven remedies; and chat rooms where information, personal experiences, and concerns are shared. Try to stick to the sites recommended by the Arthritis Foundation or fibromyalgia organizations. Don't try any unproven therapeutic approach unless you discuss it with a doctor.

CIRCUMSTANCES THAT WARRANT
SPECIAL CONSIDERATION

When fibromyalgia attacks a child or an older individual or is present during pregnancy, consider the advice provided in the following section.

Dealing with fibromyalgia in children and adolescents

Phillip was 10 when he complained of pain in his legs. The pediatrician thought it was growing pains and reassured Phillip's mother. When it persisted, X-rays of the painful areas and blood tests were done—both were normal. Ultimately, Phillip was referred to a pediatric rheumatologist, who found tender points in his knees, upper back and neck, and buttock regions. Dr. Park diagnosed Phillip as having juvenile fibromyalgia. He was started on ibuprofen. Phillip's mother went to the school and arranged for him to have a ground-level locker, made sure that his teachers noticed when his knapsack was too heavy, and checked that Phillip always attached the pack to his back. She also met with Coach Adams and showed him the types of exercises the rheumatologist recommended and the ones Phillip should avoid. Phillip was concerned that his friends would single him out for ridicule in view of his special needs, but the sixth-grade teachers handled the situation so deftly that none of his classmates really noticed.

As reviewed in Chapter 16, fibromyalgia is extremely uncommon in children. As a result, they often feel alone. Ask them to explain their pain. Make sure it's not a "growing pain" or early juvenile rheumatoid arthritis. Is reflex sympathetic dystrophy part of the syndrome? If so, this mandates a comprehensive rehabilitation program.

At school, don't let teachers accuse the child of being lazy. Educate them about the syndrome. Make things easier for the child. Have the child use a knapsack that balances weight properly. Allow and encourage the use of markers or felt-tipped pens, which make writing easier. Don't stigmatize the child. Talk to the physical education instructor. Use colorful splints if needed. Ask the child what he or she thinks will be helpful at school and at home. Children are often afraid to verbalize their concerns.

Adolescents with fibromyalgia may be noncompliant in taking medications that alter mood, behavior, or appearance. All too often, doctors are unaware of this. Teenage girls often mistake menstrual symptoms for those of fibromyalgia. Adolescents need a role model apart from the immediate family to help them through difficult times. Whether the teen turns to a relative, coach, teacher, or clergyman, encourage this type of interaction. Talk to school officials and teachers. Encourage participation in extracurricular activities that don't aggravate fibromyalgia and allow the development of self-esteem and self-respect. Wrestling is out, but the school newspaper or yearbook, French club, or drama club are possible.

Fibromyalgia and pregnancy

Ellen had mild fibromyalgia controlled with intermittent Elavil when she learned that her first child was on its way. After consulting the *Physicians Desk Reference (PDR)* in a bookstore, she stopped taking amitriptyline (Elavil). After several weeks, Ellen was in agony; her muscles and joints were stiff and achy. Dr. Rose told her to take acetaminophen (Tylenol) for the aches and acquainted her with literature suggesting that Elavil was safe during pregnancy. After she delivered a healthy daughter, Ellen's fibromyalgia flared again as a result of nightly feedings that deprived her of sleep. Every time she carried her daughter, Ellen winced in pain. She had stopped taking Elavil so that she could breast-feed, but Dr. Rose made her aware of literature showing that the immunologic protective advantages of breast-feeding do not extend beyond the first 3 months of life. Ellen occasionally took Tylenol for 3 months and weaned the baby so that she could go back on Elavil when necessary. Her husband was now able to help with the feedings, and Dr. Rose showed Ellen how to carry the baby so that minimal stress was put on her upper back muscles.

To our surprise, every year a patient of ours undergoes a therapeutic abortion because she believes that pregnancy has made her fibromyalgia too painful or that she will not be able to care for the baby. Some patients have told me that it would be impossible to get by without their medication and that they worry about its effects on the unborn.

What really happens during pregnancy? Pregnancy can aggravate fibromyalgia, but this happens only 20–30 percent of the time. Problems are associated more with sleep deprivation, hormonal changes, breast enlargement producing myofascial discomfort, morning stiffness, leg cramps, and low back pain, especially during the last trimester. Fatigue also can be a major problem. Yet, most of our patients do rather well and view these problems as worthwhile inconveniences considering the fulfillment of having a child. Even though manufacturers cannot guarantee successful pregnancies if their drugs are used, and routinely place warnings in the *PDR*, studies suggest that pregnant women can take acetaminophen (Tylenol), tricyclic antidepressants such as Elavil or Flexeril, and specific serotonin reuptake inhibitors such as Prozac in the usual doses without worrying.

Sometimes fibromyalgia flares after delivery, especially if it is associated with postpartum depression. If medication is needed, be prepared to stop breast-feeding early or do not breast-feed at all. This gives the doctor greater flexibility in recommending medication. Carry the baby in a way that straddles the weight so as not to produce too much myofascial tension. Have the spouse handle some nighttime feedings to minimize sleep disruption. If financially feasible, consider hiring someone to help with baby care and housework. Many communities have mommy's-helpers programs through churches or community centers. The temporary inconveniences caused by pregnancy should be viewed as minor nuisances on a road that ultimately yields tremendous dividends!

Fibromyalgia in the elderly

As time passed, people saw less of Frances. She started to miss bridge games and thought of excuses not to have lunch with her friends. Frances told them she was too tired and achy, the weather was bad, or she had a doctor's appointment. Her fibromyalgia medication was no longer being taken regularly, and Frances showed less enjoyment of life and decreased interest in interacting with friends. Frances's daughter accompanied her on her next doctor's visit and explained her concerns to Dr. Frank. He put Frances on nortriptyline (Pamelor), a tricyclic, in a dose also used to treat depression. Frances's daughter made sure that her mother would no longer be able to isolate herself. Within weeks she hurt less and slept better, and her old personality started to come back.

Fibromyalgia rarely develops in older patients for the first time, but as patients with the syndrome age, their problems grow. In addition to all the considerations previously noted in this chapter, there are a few additional points that warrant discussion.

First, some of the concerns we expressed about social isolation, communication skills, and community interactions need to be emphasized in elderly people. Once older persons cut themselves off from social outlets and stay indoors, their fibromyalgia worsens and their ability to function independently is impaired. Make sure that your senior citizen friend, colleague, or relative remains a viable member of the community. Also, doctors tend to put elderly patients on more medication. Whether they help the heart, blood pressure, lung, prostate, or diabetes, many of these agents interfere with fibromyalgia preparations. Some can worsen sexual performance; others can cause depression, promote aching or fatigue, or interfere with the ability to get around by producing lightheadedness or dizziness. Ask a doctor how any newly prescribed drug will influence fibromyalgia or interact with other medications given for particular health problems.

Older individuals need less sleep but are more affected by sleep medications, which produce dizziness or mental clouding. The development of osteoarthritis and osteoporosis with age tends to blur the distinction between fibromyalgia and another musculoskeletal diagnosis. Work with the family, community, and doctor to make the golden years truly golden.

SUMMING UP

Fibromyalgia patients frequently express feelings of anger, guilt, anxiety, and depression, which also aggravate the disease. There are ways to channel these feelings constructively, improve coping, relieve stress, devise positive goals, and assume favorable attitudes to make things better. Develop strategies, priorities, and organization, along with a support system of family, friends, co-workers, and the community, to stand up to the challenge of fibromyalgia.

Part VII

MEDICINES AND OTHER THERAPIES USED FOR FIBROMYALGIA

Surely every medicine is an innovation; and he that will not apply new remedies must expect new evils; for time is the greatest innovation.

Francis Bacon (1561–1626)

In the previous section, environmental influences that patients can control, such as their household and diet, were discussed. Physical and mental modalities allowing improved uses of resources and promoting the ability to cope better with fibromyalgia were also covered. In spite of these interventions, many patients also benefit from medication. The next three chapters review drugs that clearly work for fibromyalgia, those that help fibromyalgia-associated symptoms such as irritable bowel or headache, and those that have not been adequately studied but are nevertheless used by some patients. Agents that do not work or should be avoided also are mentioned.

21

Medicines That Work for Fibromyalgia

The best practitioners give to their patients the least medicine.

Frederick Saunders (1807–1902)

Nobody likes to take medicine. Many fibromyalgia patients, in particular, prefer to treat their condition with natural remedies, and many are reluctant to take prescribed medication. This problem is made more difficult because many of the most helpful preparations are designated as antidepressants. Some patients become concerned that this might create a stigma. "If you really believe what I am saying, and are convinced that I am not crazy, why are you giving me an antidepressant or antianxiety drug?" is a question we frequently hear. This problem is compounded when some insurance companies refuse to reimburse patients for these preparations, claiming that they are uncovered "psychiatric benefits."

Management of fibromyalgia includes medications from four separate families or groups, in which at least one agent has been shown in double-blinded, controlled trials (where some of the study subjects get placebo, or sugar pills) to be effective in fibromyalgia patients. These four families are (1) nonsteroidal anti-inflammatory agents (NSAIDs), (2) tricyclics, (3) specific serotonin reuptake inhibitors, and (4) benzodiazepines. The rationale for using these drugs in treating fibromyalgia is reviewed in this chapter, but first the scientific logic behind putting these drugs on our "A" list will be discussed.

THE BURDEN OF PROOF

How is a drug shown to be effective in managing a disorder?

In the United States, the Food and Drug Administration (FDA) approves drugs for specific indications. It takes many years and many dollars for an agent to be approved for a specific use, and since fibromyalgia was not recognized as a disorder until 1990, no drugs currently have FDA approval for the condition.

Many of the remedies purported to help fibromyalgia are beyond the FDA's regulatory control. These include a variety of vitamins and agents that are licensed as food supplements. As a result, promising preparations such as DHEA and melatonin (reviewed in Chapter 22) are widely available without a prescription and are being taken by patients even though few controlled trials have documented their safety or efficacy. For example, there is no legal obligation to prove that a 3-mg tablet of melatonin really contains 3 mg. Also, each batch of medication can be mixed with varying preservatives, which may affect its delivery, or bioavailability. Some of our patients have no difficulty taking the medication but react to its packaging.

Physicians who manage fibromyalgia patients must rely on scientific studies showing that a drug is effective in alleviating a particular condition. These studies use different levels of proof. When a remedy is thought to be potentially helpful for a condition it was not designed or created for, a physician usually submits a *case report* to a medical journal. Journals recognized by a committee under the direction of the National Library of Medicine in Bethesda, Maryland, as having high *peer review* standards are listed in *Index Medicus* and are also available for on-line reference. These journals evaluate all materials submitted to them by physicians, allied health professionals, or basic science experts. Papers that meet a certain standard are considered for publication, usually after the editors make comments or constructive suggestions to improve the submission. The rigor of the review and the quality of material submitted to a publication are in turn interpreted by physicians who decide to subscribe to or read the journal or ask their local medical library to obtain it. For example, the *New England Journal of Medicine* accepts less than 10 percent of the manuscripts submitted to it for publication, whereas other journals' acceptance rate can be as high as 70 percent. *Articles appearing in medical journals not recognized by the National Library of Medicine should create a healthy skepticism in the reader's mind.* For instance, if the breakthrough being claimed was so dramatic, why wouldn't a peer-reviewed, recognized journal publish it?

If a compelling case report on the effectiveness of a specific treatment for a disorder is published, it is usually followed by case reports or a series of cases. In other words, practitioners like to see that an approach is helpful in more than one patient, hopefully in more than one institution or office setting. If a large number of patients feel better when taking a drug in an *open-label* fashion (where they know what they are receiving), investigators usually design a drug trial. The complexity of drug trials varies considerably; some of the options available to an investigator are as follows:

1. *Retrospective trial*—the experiences of all patients who took a drug previously in a particular setting are analyzed.
2. *Prospective trial*—a study is initiated before the drug's use is started and the drug is evaluated as time goes on.
3. *Controlled trial*—study patients are compared with a group of individuals not getting the drug. They can be matched by race, ethnicity, age, socioeconomic level, geography, or other variables.
4. *Blinded trial*—patients do not know what they are getting, but their doctors

do. Patients are given a lot of personal attention in a drug trial and thus may feel better even though they are given a placebo; this must be factored into any study.

5. *Double-blinded trial*—neither the patients nor the doctors know if they are getting the drug or a placebo.
6. *Multicenter trial*—the study is conducted in several locations.

The most convincing results are obtained when a double-blinded, international, multicenter, prospective, placebo-controlled trial using a large number of patients demonstrates a drug's ameliorative effects.

How do patients decide which drug to try for fibromyalgia?

Popular publications such as *Good Housekeeping*, *Time*, and the *Reader's Digest* frequently address health-related topics and generally provide a balanced overview. Additionally, anybody who accesses the Internet and types in "fibromyalgia" as a keyword will find numerous references for a variety of remedies. Many of these are unproven and are promoted by individuals or companies that want to make money from naive patients who do not feel well and will try anything that seems harmless and inexpensive. Other media such as television, radio, videocassettes, and street or store advertising market a variety of remedies that claim to help fibromyalgia. The next three chapters offer an overview of most of these and place them in their proper perspective.

WHICH DRUGS CLEARLY HELP FIBROMYALGIA?

Are NSAIDs and aspirin beneficial?

NSAIDs and aspirin block the actions of a chemical known as *prostaglandin*, which is responsible for some of the pain and inflammation of arthritis. Most fibromyalgia patients are familiar with these preparations, which are listed in Table 11. Preparations such as Advil, Aleve, or Orudis KT are available without a prescription.

Although these drugs are not dramatically effective in managing fibromyalgia, placebo-controlled, double-blinded trials have shown that ibuprofen (the active ingredient of Advil and Motrin) and naproxen (Naprosyn, Aleve, Naprelan) in combination with other fibromyalgia remedies decrease pain in patients with the syndrome. They also alleviate premenstrual syndrome complaints, joint aches, and headaches. Doctors managing fibromyalgia patients recommend that these agents be used in any of several ways. First, they may be used on an occasional as-needed basis for pain breakthroughs. In this instance, blood counts need to be checked once or twice a year. Second, an NSAID may be prescribed on an ongoing, regular basis. In this case, patients should visit their doc-

Table 11. *Major NSAIDs*

Salicylates
    Aspirin
    Sodium salicylates (Trilisate, Disalcid)
    Diflusinal (Dolobid)
    Magnesium salicylate (Magan, Doan's)
Propionic acid derivatives
    Oxaprozin (Daypro)
    Naproxen (Naprosyn, Anaprox, Aleve)
    Flurbiprofen (Ansaid)
    Ibuprofen (Motrin, Advil, Mediprin, Nuprin)
    Ketoprofen (Orudis KT, Orudis, Oruvail)
    Fenoprofen (Nalfon)
Acetic acid derivatives
    Sulindac (Clinoril)
    Diclofenac (Voltaren, Cataflam, Arthrotec)
    Tolmetin (Tolectin)
    Indomethacin (Indocin)
Others
    Etodolac (Lodine)
    Ketrolac (Toradol)
    Piroxicam (Feldene)
    Nabumetone (Relafen)
    Meclofenamate (Meclomen, Ponstel)

tor every 3 to 4 months and have laboratory testing, including a blood count, and liver and kidney function screening. Third, pharmacists are now making NSAIDs as gels or salves (particularly diclofenac and ketoprofen) that can be applied to painful areas. Aspirin-containing preparations such as Ben-Gay have been available for some time.

NSAIDs and aspirin are not without side effects. Patients who take these agents on a regular basis may experience fluid retention, bloating, upset stomach, diarrhea, or constipation. Ongoing administration requires checking patients for gastrointestinal ulcers, liver and kidney function, and rashes. In the United States, 3 percent of regular NSAID users annually have gastrointestinal bleeds, often necessitating hospitalization.

Why do doctors prescribe tricyclic antidepressants and other similar antidepressants?

How do tricyclics work?

Tricyclic antidepressants (TCAs) have been available for more than 40 years and represent the old, reliable approach to managing fibromyalgia. In doses lower than those demonstrated to alleviate depression, TCAs have a variety of beneficial effects on the syndrome. First, they may increase the amount of delta wave sleep. Second, they improve the availability of serotonin to nerve cells. Third, they heighten the effect of endorphins, which decreases pain. Finally, they relax muscles. These actions are accomplished by the combined effect of increasing levels of serotonin, dopamine, and norepinephrine, acting as an antihistamine and decreasing parasympathetic ANS activity. TCAs are not addictive, have no narcotic effect, and only indirectly decrease pain.

Which tricyclic should be used?

Sarah had mild fibromyalgia but tried to avoid taking medication because she was very sensitive to anything she took. However, the Vermont winter had been particularly cold and damp, and there was a lot of tumult at her company, Archer Industries, which created more than the usual amount of stress. Dr. Craig prescribed cyclobenzaprine (Flexeril), but after taking a half tablet 2 hours before bedtime, Sarah felt like a zombie for part of the next day. Dr. Craig changed to nortriptyline (Pamelor), which made her mouth so dry that she had to get up several times during the night to drink water. Next, trazodone (Desyrel) therapy was given, which helped Sarah sleep but did not relieve her painful spasms. Finally, Dr. Craig recommended using liquid doxepin (Sinequan) drops, which made Sarah sleep and relieved her muscle pain and spasms.

Numerous TCA preparations are available to treat fibromyalgia, but as in Sarah's case, it often takes several attempts before the right dose and preparation are found for that individual. The most commonly used TCAs are listed in Table 12. The most commonly used preparation is *amitriptyline hydrochloride* (Elavil or Endep). Elavil is available as a 10-, 25-, 50-, 75-, or 100-mg tablet. Practitioners treating depression prescribe at least 25 mg a day, and 50–150 mg a day is probably a more effective dose. However, as little as 10 mg can decrease pain, relax muscles, and promote restful sleep. Since Elavil takes 2–3 hours to work, we advise most of our patients to take it several hours before going to sleep. Elavil usually lasts for about 8 hours once it starts to work. Hence, if it is taken right at bedtime, one can have a "hangover"—a drugged feeling persisting into the midmorning hours. The beneficial effects of Elavil may not be fully evident for 3–6 weeks. We tend to prescribe doses of 10–25 mg at night. Some patients are very sensitive to TCAs. In these instances, we prescribe *doxepin hydrochloride* (Sinequan or Adapin) since doses as low as 3 mg can be derived from the liquid suspension. Doxepin dosing is the same as with Elavil, but for unclear reasons, doses of over 25 mg tend to promote considerable weight gain; as a result, we usually start with Elavil.

Cyclobenzaprine (Flexeril) is not marketed for depression and is approved by the FDA as a muscle relaxant. Consequently, we use this agent for patients with

Table 12. *Medication families clearly effective in treating fibromyalgia*

Tricyclic and closely related antidepressant preparations (TCAs)
    Amitriptyline hydrochloride (Elavil, Endep)
    Imipramine hydrochloride (Janimine, Tofranil)
    Doxepin hydrochloride (Adapin, Sinequan)
    Nortriptyline hydrochloride (Aventyl, Pamelor)
    Desipramine hydrochloride (Norpramin, Petrofane)
    Trazodone hydrochloride (Desyrel)
    Cyclobenzaprine hydrochloride (Flexeril)
Specific serotonin reuptake inhibitors (SSRIs)
    Fluoxetine hydrochloride (Prozac)
    Sertraline hydrochloride (Zoloft)
    Paroxetine hydrochloride (Paxil)
Combination TCA-SSRI preparations
    Venlafaxine hydrochloride (Effexor)
    Nafazodone (Serzone)
Benzodiazepines and closely related drugs
    Clonazepam (Klonopin)
    Diazepam (Valium)
    Chlordiazepoxide (Librium)
    Alprazolam (Xanax)

---

prominent musculoskeletal problems and few, if any, psychological problems. Its prescription also eliminates the stigma attached to taking an antidepressant. In our experience, 10 mg of cyclobenzaprine is equivalent to 15–25 mg of doxepin, and its actions are quite similar. We often advise patients to cut the tablet in half or even in quarters. Controlled studies repeatedly have documented the effectiveness of doxepin and cyclobenzaprine in managing fibromyalgia.

Certain patients have slightly different needs. For example, when depression is prominent, we tend to use *nortriptyline hydrochloride* (Aventyl, Pamelor), *imipramine hydrochloride* (Tofranil, Janimine), or *desipramine hydrochloride* (Norpramin, Petrofane) in Elavil-like doses, but we usually prescribe at least 50 mg in the evening. Patients who have more of a sleep problem and less of a pain problem often derive benefit from *trazodone hydrochloride* (Desyrel) in doses ranging from 50 to 200 mg at bedtime.

What are the side effects of TCAs?

The toxicity of TCAs varies considerably. The way they are broken down, or *metabolized*, varies as much as 50-fold among patients. The most common side effect is drowsiness, although 10–15 percent of patients have a "reverse reaction" and become energetic after taking the medication. In these instances TCAs can be taken in the morning, but the sensation may be unpleasant to some patients and we usually stop the drug when this happens. Occasionally we might try another TCA, but if the patient complains of agitation or twitching, this is usually a signal to switch to a different family of drugs. Although dry mouth, blurred vision, constipation, low blood pressure, and palpitations are the most common side effects of TCAs, manufacturers list several hundred rare reactions to these agents in the *PDR*. Many of these side effects can be ameliorated by lowering the dose or switching to a different preparation. Weight gain, fluid retention, and bloating tend to occur in antidepressant doses but are uncommon in fibromyalgia doses. Cyclobenzaprine and trazodone produce these complications least often.

TCAs should be used very carefully, if at all, in young children (under the age of 12), in patients who are pregnant or breast-feeding, and in elderly people who might become confused in the middle of the night. For instance, when older patients are dizzy, sleepy, and have poor balance, they could fall and fracture an osteoporotic hip when they get up to go to the bathroom.

Sometimes, the effects of TCAs wear off with time. "Drug holidays," or weeks without using them or temporarily switching to a different TCA, can restore their effectiveness.

How much medication should a patient take and for how long?

As we've noted, fibromyalgia patients generally don't like to take medicine, and few doctors will prescribe TCAs if patients think they must be taken forever. In fact, this need not be. We usually reevaluate our patients 1 month after starting a TCA. If their responses are favorable, the TCA is continued in a full dose for 3–6 months. At that point, we usually taper the drug to every other night and ultimately advise the patient to use it as needed. In other words, when a good night's sleep is critical, when it's been a particularly stressful time, when premenstrual symptoms are present, or if the weather has changed, a few nights on a TCA can be helpful. We have found that several months on a TCA tends to reset one's "pain thermostat," or threshold, and long-term use of the drug is frequently not needed. A summary of several published studies suggests that TCAs alone lead to a significant improvement in one-third of fibromyalgia patients and some improvement in another third after 6 months of treatment.

What do we do if the patient feels only somewhat better or does not respond at all? The sections that follow review other options.

What about specific serotonin reuptake inhibitors?

Amanda had an excellent response to Flexeril at first, but after several months it became apparent that this was not enough. She still developed spasms and at times was too tired to function at the accustomed level for the medical office she managed. Dr. Smith prescribed low-dose fluoxetane (Prozac). This made her less anxious, diminished her pain, and provided an energy boost but also eliminated her libido and caused her to break out in cold sweats for no apparent reason several times a week. Dr. Smith switched her to sertraline (Zoloft), which did not work as well and gave her headaches. Finally, paroxetine (Paxil) was tried in addition to the Flexeril. It allowed Amanda to function normally at work, minimized her pain, and had no adverse effects. After 3 months on Paxil she discontinued it, without any problems, and continues to do well.

Specific serotonin reuptake inhibitors (SSRIs) are the new kids on the block. Available since the mid-1980s, these drugs have revolutionized our management of depression. The use of these agents in fibromyalgia is a two-edged sword. *When taken by themselves (without a TCA or benzodiazepine), SSRIs can potentially make fibromyalgia worse.* Why? By promoting the release of serotonin, SSRIs reduce fatigue and increase energy. This, in turn, can make it harder to sleep at night, which may aggravate fibromyalgia. As a result, early studies using SSRIs in fibromyalgia produced negative results. It was not until these agents were tested in *combination* with TCAs that it became clear that SSRIs can provide greater improvement in fibromyalgia than TCAs alone.

SSRIs are used to manage the fatigue, cognitive impairment, and depression associated with fibromyalgia and can modestly alleviate pain by promoting the release of endorphins. They usually become effective within 2–3 weeks. SSRIs are not habit-forming and contain no narcotics. Also, as with TCAs, very low doses are often therapeutic; these doses are much lower than those used for depression. Patients with fibromyalgia are often very sensitive to all types of medication.

Available agents include the SSRI prototype, fluoxetane hydrochloride (Prozac). Since Prozac is available in 10- and 20-mg doses, and as a liquid suspension that can deliver as little as a few milligrams, we tend to start our patients at 5–20 mg a day in the morning. Prozac is stronger than other SSRIs and produces more agitation, sweating, nausea, and palpitations. SSRIs can also help anxiety disorders and are now FDA approved for obsessive-compulsive behavior. Some patients have reported weight gain (only 20 percent lose weight) and decreased libido while using Prozac; second-line agents may be helpful if these side effects occur.

Physicians also can prescribe two "kinder, gentler" Prozacs—sertraline hydrochloride (Zoloft) and paroxetine hydrochloride (Paxil)—particularly for those with milder disease or a greater tendency toward drug side effects. The usual doses are 50–200 mg a day for Zoloft and 10–60 mg a day for Paxil. Recently, two combination TCA-SSRIs have become available: venlafaxine hydrochloride (Effexor) and nafazodone (Serzone). Although these preparations are very effective for depression, their use can be confusing in fibromyalgia since their effects on sleep are highly variable and must be monitored carefully.

As with TCAs, we try to use SSRIs for only a few months and let the body's pain and energy thermostat reset itself. After several months, we have found that SSRIs can reduce cognitive dysfunction and fatigue without disrupting sleep patterns, and these agents often can be used without TCAs.

Benzodiazepines: They work, but use them with extreme caution!

Shelly could not tolerate any of the TCAs Dr. Ray prescribed for fibromyalgia because they "wired" her and caused tremors. Her major problem was an inability to sleep, and her legs would not stay still at night. A neurologist who was consulted advised trying clonazepam (Klonopin) at bedtime. Its effect was dramatic. Not only was she able to sleep without interruption, but her musculoskeletal aches disappeared and Shelly felt like a new person. However, after 6 months, she realized that two Klonopin pills were needed when she had previously gotten by with one. Shelly also began to cry without provocation, which was downright embarrassing. Dr. Ray tapered and then stopped the Klonopin for a month. He told Shelly that she could take it only occasionally and prescribed another sleep aid for regular use.

Benzodiazepines relieve fibromyalgia symptoms primarily by eliminating the abnormal brain waves that produce the alpha-delta sleep wave abnormality and by decreasing sleep myoclonus, or restless legs syndrome. Approved by the FDA for use in epilepsy, a condition characterized by abnormal electrical impulses in the brain, these agents clearly have a place in selected patients with fibromyalgia. Additionally, benzodiazepines are tranquilizers that promote relaxation and unspasm muscles. Their action is mediated by increasing serotonin and inhibiting transmission of excitatory nerve impulses in the brain or spinal cord via increasing levels of the neurotransmitter termed gamma aminobutyric acid (GABA). Double-blind, controlled studies have established their efficacy in treating the restless legs syndrome and anxiety associated with fibromyalgia. *However, benzodiazepines must be used very carefully because they may be addicting and in a small minority of patients cause a serious depression that lasts until the drug is stopped.*

The principal agent used in fibromyalgia is *clonazepam* (Klonopin). One of the best drugs for epilepsy, twitching, restless legs syndrome, or jerking sensations, Klonopin, when given for fibromyalgia in doses of 0.5- to 1.5 mg at bedtime, promotes restful sleep and relaxes the muscles. It does little if anything for pain. It is a long-acting drug and may produce a morning hangover. It is otherwise well tolerated, with few side effects, the most common being fatigue and diarrhea. The effects of Klonopin decrease with time and the drug can be addicting after as little as several weeks of use.

Table 13. *Dr. Wallace's approach to fibromyalgia therapies*

1. Give the patient a firm diagnosis, provide education about the disease, review physical measures and lifestyle approaches.
2. For 50 percent of patients we also prescribe medication. We tell them to use intermittent NSAIDs and start a TCA.
   a. One-third have an excellent response to the TCA, and many stop taking it within 6 months or use it intermittently.
   b. One-third need ongoing therapy with a TCA, with or without the addition of an SSRI.
   c. One-third have no response to TCAs or SSRIs and need other approaches.
3. One-third of patients benefit from an SSRI added to a TCA. Half of this group can discontinue the SSRI within 6 months.
4. One-sixth of patients are given SSRI-TCA combinations with benzodiazepines. Nearly half of this group ultimately report substantial relief.
5. One-sixth of patients have severe, resistant fibromyalgia and require additional aggressive measures and therapies.

When should one use Klonopin? We prescribe it for patients who cannot tolerate TCAs or have a suboptimal response to a combination of TCAs and SSRIs. Additionally, we use Klonopin for restless legs syndrome and to relieve acute steroid withdrawal symptoms. However, we advise our patients to take the drug only for 2 weeks at first. If additional or continued use is needed, we often ask them to take it every other night so that its effects will not wear off and it cannot be habit-forming. About 10 percent of the time, our patients develop severe, sudden depression. If this occurs, we stop the drug over several days and the depression subsides within a few days. Benzodiazepines can be administered with TCAs or SSRIs, and the combination may be useful.

Other drugs in the benzodiazepine family may be helpful. The much maligned *diazepam* (Valium) also can be addicting and can cause depression. However, we occasionally use it for severe muscle spasms, for patients who want a Klonopin-like drug at night that is shorter-acting, and for the 10 percent of fibromyalgia patients who have balance disturbances or dizziness. Valium is the drug of choice for benign positional vertigo, a syndrome brought on when changing positions causes dizziness, which can be an autonomic symptom of fibromyalgia. *Chlordiazepoxide* (Librium) has similar actions. Controlled studies have shown that it is particularly helpful for preventing convulsions in acute alcohol withdrawal and in irritable bowel syndrome (functional bowel disease) as the Librium-containing preparation Librax. Approximately 10–30 percent of fibromyalgia patients have anxiety, which may warrant treatment with medication. A controlled study conducted by Jon Russell at the University of Texas at San Antonio clearly showed that *alprazolam* (Xanax), in doses of 0.5–1.5 mg a day, decreases fibromyalgia-associated anxiety. Xanax should never be stopped suddenly. When no longer needed, it can be tapered slowly over several weeks.

SUMMING UP

We frequently encounter patients who are so grateful to finally have a diagnosis explaining their symptoms and signs that, once they have read about fibromyalgia, they tell us that they will learn to live with it. Indeed, if the physical and emotional measures reviewed in Chapters 18 and 19 are accepted, as many as half of all fibromyalgia patients in a community practice do not need any ongoing medication. Many of our patients take an occasional Advil and Aleve for pain during the day or Flexeril at night when they are stressed out or hurt more than usual. Despite this, at least 50 percent of our fibromyalgia patients are started on at least a TCA. One-third of them have a spectacular response, and many are able to stop the drug after several months and thereafter use it only occasionally. Another third require the addition of an SSRI or a benzodiazepine, which leads to some improvement. Another third (or one-sixth of all fibromyalgia patients) do not respond satisfactorily to any of these measures. Some of the preparations discussed in the next two chapters are then prescribed, and this subgroup of patients usually benefits from psychotherapy given as an adjunct to physical measures and medication. Tables 12 and 13 summarize these concepts.

22

Drugs That Are Useful in Selected Fibromyalgia Patients

Life as we find it is too hard for us; it entails too much pain,
too many disappointments, impossible tasks. We cannot do
without palliative remedies.

Sigmund Freud (1856–1939),
Civilization and Its Discontents, 1930

Doctors often prescribe drugs for fibromyalgia patients with distinct manifestations associated with the disorder such as tension headache, chronic fatigue, or bladder spasms. Few of the preparations discussed in this chapter have been shown to be specifically effective in fibromyalgia, but nearly all of them are widely prescribed by doctors who treat fibromyalgia patients. This chapter reviews our clinical experience with these drugs for fibromyalgia-related manifestations and presents a personalized, critical evaluation of them.

LOCALIZED REMEDIES

Do tender point injections work?

One of the most commonly employed interventions in fibromyalgia is the *tender point injection*. Controlled studies have clearly demonstrated its usefulness in patients with myofascial pain syndrome. When a patient comes to our office and reports that a specific point—for example, in the upper back or neck area—hurts, we try to ascertain how severe this discomfort is in relation to their overall pain. If we are told that at least 30 percent (and preferably more than 50 percent) of their pain at the moment is from a specific tender area, this is an indication for a local injection. Patients who "hurt all over" rarely respond to tender point injections for more than a few days.

Once we have decided to give a local injection or injections (usually limiting the number of injections to three per visit, with visits spaced several weeks apart), what preparations are used? The drugs of choice always include a local pain deadener, or anesthetic, usually xylocaine, novocaine, or marcaine. After the painful area is sprayed with a coolant anesthetic such as ethyl chloride or fluori-methane, the anesthetic in the shots usually works immediately. Sometimes a steroid is added to the anesthetic in the same syringe.

Not all doctors use steroids for tender point injections. However, the doses we use are very low, and systemic effects are uncommon. The recommended preparations include triamcinolone (Kenalog or Aristocort), which is the most useful but must be given carefully since it sometimes dissolves fat tissue around the injection site and leaves a "pit"; betamethasone (Celestone), which is quite effective but burns more than other brands; methylprednisolone (Depo-Medrol), which does not last as long as the others but is well tolerated; and dexamethasone (Decadron LA), which is mild and well tolerated. The full benefits of these injections are usually apparent within several days, although patients may complain of local pain, flushing, or tingling for the first 1 or 2 days. The physician has to be very careful when injecting the upper back areas. He or she usually grasps or "lifts up" an area of fat or fascia to avoid puncturing the lung, a temporarily painful condition known as a *pneumothorax*. Pneumothorax is the most critical complication of the procedure, although it is very rare. Local injections can be given as often as needed, but we have found them worthwhile only if they provide relief for at least several weeks.

Figure 22 illustrates a tender point injection.

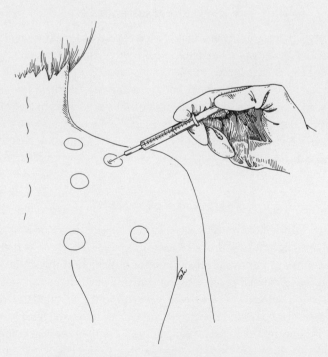

Fig. 22 *Example of a tender point injection*

Do nerve blocks or epidurals work?

Nerve blocks are anesthetics and/or steroids injected into nerve tissues to relieve pain. Severe, localized, painful manifestations of reflex sympathetic dystrophy respond to nerve blocks, especially in the stellate ganglion area of the shoulder region.

Many patients with regional myofascial pain are incorrectly diagnosed as having herniated discs or arthritic disorders of the spine on the basis of abnormal X-rays, CT scans, or MRI scans. Unless an EMG with a nerve conduction study confirms that these abnormalities are producing physiologic changes, these X-ray or scanning results should be viewed with some skepticism. A recent study of healthy, asymptomatic people in their 40s who volunteered to have spinal MRI scans showed that 30 percent of them had significant abnormalities that rarely if ever caused symptoms. We have many fibromyalgia and myofascial pain syndrome patients who received epidural spinal nerve blocks for nonspecific radiographic abnormalities and localized symptoms that mimicked a disc disorder. The steroid in these epidural blocks often worsens the symptoms of fibromyalgia (see Chapter 13). Nerve blocks are usually prescribed only if there is clear evidence of a herniated disc or a degenerative process called *spinal stenosis*.

When are local salves used?

Topical gels, creams, ointments, and lotions have been used to treat local pain. Believe it or not, agents containing *capsaicin* (Zostrix, Dolorac) are cayenne pepper derivatives that locally deplete substance P (a pain neurotransmitter). These preparations frequently burn but are otherwise harmless and take a week or so to work. Give yourself the rheumatologist's version of the "Pepsi challenge"! Apply capsaicin for 1 week to one side of the body and see if it feels better than the other side. Other local preparations include *topical NSAIDs and aspirin* (see Chapter 21).

MUSCLE RELAXANTS

In an effort to minimize muscle spasms and muscle pain, doctors prescribe a variety of muscle-relaxing drugs. However, unlike TCAs or benzodiazepines, these agents have little or no effect on endorphins, pain threshold levels, pain perception, or emotional reactions, and only modest effects on sleep patterns. Nevertheless, in selected patients who have difficulty taking TCAs or who are not candidates for benzodiazepines, we sometimes prescribe muscle relaxants.

When muscle relaxants were first introduced, they were revolutionary and were frequently abused by patients and doctors. In the 1960s, use of the muscle relaxant *meprobamate* (Milltown) was widespread, but the agent fell into disfavor when it was found to be highly addictive. A milder form of meprobamate, *carisoprodol* (Soma; Soma Compound contains aspirin), has become one of the most widely prescribed muscle relaxants in the United States. It acts on the nerves to relax muscles rather than on the muscles themselves. A double-blind, controlled trial suggested that Soma decreases pain, improves sleep quality, and increases the sense of well-being in fibromyalgia patients.

Preparations similar to Soma are also popular. All of these agents can produce fatigue and dull the senses a bit, and none of them should be used with alcohol. They are primarily prescribed for patients with acute low back pain or whiplash-induced spasm without fibromyalgia and are not intended for long-term use. An agent that unspasms muscles while promoting wakefulness is Norgesic Forte, a combination of aspirin, caffeine, and *orphenadrine citrate* (a muscle relaxant). Ophenadine is also available without the aspirin and caffeine as Norflex. Other widely used preparations include *methocarbamol* (Robaxisal with aspirin, Robaxin without aspirin), *chloroxazone* (Parafon), and *metaxalone (*Skelaxin).

As noted in Chapter 5, magnesium plays a central role in muscle contraction. An interesting preparation containing *magnesium and malic acid* (available as Super Malate and Fibroplex, among other names) is available from health food stores. Controlled studies from England and Texas in peer-reviewed journals have documented modest effects of this preparation on muscle spasm, fatigue, and pain in fibromyalgia. If patients take a dose larger than that recommended on the bottle (two very large pills three times a day), its effects become apparent within a week; side effects are uncommon. This combination may work as a result of interactions between magnesium and calcium channels within muscles and the generation of adenosine triphosphate (ATP), our cellular fuel. It occasionally induces diarrhea, drowsiness, lightheadedness, and dizziness at high doses.

Leg cramps are reported more commonly by fibromyalgia patients than by healthy people. They often respond to the administration of *quinine*, an old standby available since the 1600s.

PAIN KILLERS

Pain killers are analgesics that temporarily deaden the discomfort of fibromyalgia without reducing the underlying pain or its associated fatigue. Since higher and higher doses are needed after a while to maintain the same level of effectiveness, many pain killers are addicting. Narcotic preparations tend to be constipating, produce nausea, and reduce mental acuity. In one study, 36 percent of fibromyalgia patients required strong analgesics at some point in their disease course, but fewer than 5 percent needed triplicate, or controlled narcotic-containing substances.

Drugs marketed for mild to moderate pain

The safest but least effective analgesic is *acetaminophen* (Tylenol). To protect the liver and kidney, patients should never take more than six tablets a day. A modified NSAID (see Chapter 21), *ketrolac* (Toradol), is indicated for short-term use in patients with postoperative pain or severe pain flares. Toradol has been associated with kidney or liver damage and stomach ulceration if used for longer than 1 week. *Tramadol* (Ultram) is a unique preparation that raises seratonin and noradrenaline levels and blocks several pain pathways. Among these is the NMDA receptor, or excitatory amino acid pathway, which may play a role in promoting fibromyalgia pain (reviewed in Chapter 4). Some fibromyalgia patients find that taking two tablets every 4–6 hours for severe pain breaks the pain-spasm-pain cycle.

Drugs marketed for moderate to severe pain

We occasionally prescribe narcotic analgesics for short-term use (less than 1 week for acute flares) or for breakthrough pain (a few tablets a month). *Codeine* is available alone or in combination with either aspirin or acetaminophen but frequently causes nausea. *Propoxyphene* (Darvon) is similar to codeine in efficacy but is slightly weaker, and is also available in combination with aspirin (Darvon Compound) or acetaminophen (Darvocet-N). A few patients prefer the relatively nonaddicting *pentazocine* (Talwin NX or Talacen) for moderate pain.

Hydrocodone (Vicodin, with acetaminophen; or vicoprofen, with ibuprofen, Lortab) and *oxycodone* (Percodan, with aspirin; or Percocet, with acetaminophen) are very potent and highly addictive. Doctors should be on their guard if a patient requests Vicodin with Soma since this combination can produce a dangerous, addictive "high" and is sold as a street drug.

When pain becomes unbearable

Allan herniated disks in his neck and low back after a skydiving accident. Although surgery was successful in aligning the spine, he experienced excruciating pain in his neck, low back, and adjacent muscles. Allan consulted neurologists, neurosurgeons, orthopedists, and rheumatologists (two of each). He underwent three MRI scans, two CT scans, an EMG with nerve conduction study, numerous X-rays of his cervical and lumbar spine, and blood tests. Dr. Sand ultimately diagnosed him as having a postsurgical pain amplification syndrome with posttraumatic fibromyalgia. Although Allan looked healthy, without oxycodon (Percodan) and carisoprodol (Soma) he was barely able to move without screaming. Over several months, the amount of Percodan needed to make his life tolerable increased from 4 to 8 pills a day. Dr. Sand instructed Allan how to inject himself with meperidine (Demerol). The shots helped for a few hours, but the dose escalated over the following weeks. Dr. Sand referred Allan to a comprehensive pain management center. They admitted him to the hospital and gave him a 72-hour timed release narcotic patch to avoid the problems of withdrawal or craving. He was seen by a physical therapist and an occupational therapist. An anesthesiologist provided local nerve blocks and trigger point injections; a psychologist initiated biofeedback and other relaxation techniques; and a psychiatrist prescribed high doses of a TCA to make him less aware of the pain along with gabapentin (Neurontin). The doctors met for an hour once a week and coordinated Allan's care. After 3 weeks, he was discharged on tapering doses of medicines and felt better than he had in a long time.

Stronger narcotics are available in many states as a triplicate prescription, whereby copies are sent to state or federal agencies for closer monitoring. Any physician who uses triplicate preparations should have some training in pain management techniques. Only a small minority of fibromyalgia patients ever require *morphine, hydromorphine* (Dilaudid), *levorphanol* (Levo-Dromoran), or *meperidine* (Demerol). Another opioid, *methadone*, may additionally block NMDA receptors. In pain management centers, these agents are also available as timed-release patches or in pumps for severe cases. In our experience, some fibromyalgia patients who progress this far also have severe psychiatric disorders or reflex sympathetic dystrophy (see Chapter 13). Despite their potency, morphine-like drugs often fail to relieve fibromyalgia pain. Fibromyalgia patients with serious pain have the best outcome when they are managed as Allan was—at a multidisciplinary pain center employing the coordinated use of pain medications, nerve blocks, counseling, and physical rehabilitation techniques.

NERVE PAIN AND SPASM

Betty had a mild case of fibromyalgia, and treatment helped her muscle spasms and her difficulty sleeping. However, Betty felt that her nerves were "on fire." Her legs burned, felt like pins and needles, and at times seemed numb. Dr. Black ordered an MRI scan of her low back, a vascular study of her legs, blood tests, and an EMG and nerve conduction study of her muscles and nerves. They showed no evidence of a herniated disc, poor circulation, inflammation, or diabetes. Dr. Black explained that about 10 percent of her fibromyalgia patients had otherwise unexplainable severe nerve pain. She prescribed valproic acid (Depakote) and then carbamezine (Tegretol). They both helped a bit, and after several weeks Betty was switched to gabapentin (Neurontin). Betty felt worse until Dr. Black told her that Neurontin took several weeks to work and that the dose was built up slowly. Eventually, Betty noticed less nerve pain and was able to function much better.

Infrequently, patients with fibromyalgia report painful numbness, burning and tingling, or severe shooting spasms or jerks that do not respond to TCAs. Even though epilepsy is not associated with fibromyalgia, a group of agents used to manage seizures may be helpful in managing fibromyalgia complaints. These include *carbamezine* (Tegretol), *clonazepam* (Klonopin), *phenytoin* (Dilantin), *valproic acid* (Depakote), and *gabapentin* (Neurontin). As an example, Neurontin increases GABA levels, which slows down the central nervous system's nerve impulses. GABA also blocks the release of excitatory amino acids, which promote chronic pain. Patients using these agents should be followed on a regular basis, since the dosage and adjustments of these drugs should be supervised by a neurologist or another physician familiar with their uses and side effects, including monitoring of blood counts and liver tests.

Mexiletene (Mexitil) is a preparation known to be effective in managing irregular heartbeat. It is also helpful for diabetic neuropathy pain, and some of our fibromyalgia patients have had less nerve pain while taking it. *Baclofen* (Lioresal) relieves painful muscle spasms in some fibromyalgia patients by interacting with the GABA pathway (as do Valium-like drugs) to decrease spinal cord reflexes. It is usually prescribed for patients with multiple sclerosis, a condition not usually associated with fibromyalgia. A more toxic form of baclofen, *dantrolene* (Dantrium), should be avoided. Finally, a form of *L-dopa* (Sinemet) prescribed for Parkinson's disease (recognized by a shuffled walk and tremors) can successfully treat the jerks and twitches of restless legs syndrome that keep patients with fibromyalgia awake at night.

HOW CAN DRYNESS BE MANAGED?

Complaints of dry, gritty eyes and difficult tearing, decreased sweating, or a dry, hacking cough from dehydrated lungs may be reported in fibromyalgia. As reviewed in Chapter 11, some fibromyalgia patients have TCA or other drug-mediated, autonomic-based, or immune (Sjogren's syndrome) sources of dryness.

Ocular dryness (*keratoconjunctivitis sicca*) is treated symptomatically with artificial tears or by surgically closing the tear ducts. Dry mouth (*xerostomia*) is managed by drinking plenty of fluids and sucking on sour lemon drops or Lifesavers. Since frequent use of these candies can contribute to tooth decay, we advise patients to drink plain or carbonated water (seltzer, club soda) with citrus juice (orange, lime, lemon, grapefruit, tangerine) squeezed in. A variety of salivary preparations such as Salivart help relieve more severe cases. Careful attention to good dental hygiene and regular visits to the dentist reduce the risk of drying-mediated tooth decay and gum deterioration.

Lungs can be humidified with fluids that mobilize mucus, such as chicken soup and agents containing *guaifenesin* (Organidin, Humabid). Nasal dryness

symptoms are alleviated with petroleum jelly (Vaseline), skin dryness with mois-
turizing soaps (Alpha-Keri, Vaseline Intensive Care, Dove), and vaginal dryness
with lubricants (K-Y Lubricating Jelly) or hormonal vaginal (Premarin) salves or
suppositories.

From a medication standpoint, *pilocarpine* (Salagen), taken in doses of 5–10
mg every 6–8 hours, promotes parasympathetic autonomic functions such as
tearing, sweating, salivation, urinating, and defecating, which were reviewed in
Chapter 7. It also reduces vaginal dryness, which may be an annoying problem in
some patients. If the dryness has an immune basis, physicians sometimes prescribe *hydroxychloroquine* (Plaquenil). The reader is referred to the Sjogren's
Syndrome Foundation listing in Appendix 1 for more information.

DRUGS THAT IMPROVE SLEEP

Casey could not tolerate any of the TCAs given to manage her fibromyalgia. Her depression, anxiety, fatigue, and pain, however, were reduced by
fluoxetine (Prozac)—which, however, caused one problem: she was unable
to sleep. Over-the-counter sleep aids such as Sominex or Sleep-Eze simply
did not work. Casey's internist prescribed triazolam (Halcion), which put
her to sleep, but she could not remember anything for several hours when
she awakened. Clonazepam (Klonopin) also drugged her too much in the
morning. Finally, tenazepam (Restoril) was tried, which allowed Casey to
continue using Prozac and to sleep without feeling hung over.

Despite using the measures discussed in Chapter 18, some patients still have
difficulty sleeping. Occasionally, patients cannot take—or are unable to sleep in
spite of taking—TCAs, or benzodiazepines. In a controlled study, the benzodi-
azepine-related agent *zolpidem* (Ambien) promoted sleep in fibromyalgia
patients but did not relieve pain or morning stiffness. Few other sleep aids have
been studied in fibromyalgia patients. Other benzodiazepines promote restful
sleep but have little effect on the fibromyalgia. They include *florazepam* (Dal-
mane), *tenazepam* (Restoril), *oxazepam* (Serax), *quazepam* (Doral), and *estazo-
lam* (ProSom). *Diphenhydramine* (Benadryl, Tylenol PM, Sleep-eze), *dimenhy-
drinate* (Dramamine), and *meclizine* (Bonine) are antihistamines that induce
drowsiness most of the time and have no demonstrated benefits in treating fibromyalgia. In a controlled trial, a nonbenzodiazepine not available in the United
States, *zipiclone*, improved the sleep of fibromyalgia patients but did not reduce
their morning stiffness, tenderness, or pain. Some sleep specialists have had success with an herb from *valerian root* (see Table 16).

Melatonin is marketed as a food additive, but it is really a hormone made by
the pineal gland of the brain. It regulates sleep cycles, increases growth hormone
production, and increases acetylchloline release in brain cells. A 3- to 6-mg dose
promotes a shallow sleep for 4–6 hours.

Sleeping pills to avoid

Until the 1960s, when benzodiazepines became available, barbiturates were the most commonly prescribed family of sleeping pills. Benzodiazepines represented a major breakthrough and, as a result, young upstarts such as me became hypercritical of anybody who would ever use a barbiturate. When I was an internal medicine resident at Cedars-Sinai Medical Center in Los Angeles, my fellow residents and I would snicker at some of the "old-timer" attending physicians based on their notoriety. We would boast to our friends in a whisper after saying hello to one of these doctors, "He was the doctor who prescribed barbiturates to Marilyn Monroe." However, barbiturates were the only tools the old-timers had, and their toxicity was not widely appreciated at the time. In addition to contributing to the death of many talented people, barbiturates (e.g., Seconal, Nembutal, Placidyl) can be addictive, do not promote refreshing sleep, and are associated with seizures if suddenly withdrawn. They should be prescribed only by a sleep specialist, neurologist, or physician very familiar with their use. *Triazolam* (Halcion) should not be used since it has been associated with memory impairment.

WHAT CAN YOU TAKE FOR A HEADACHE?

Just as they were to Colleen in Chapter 10, headaches can be particularly disabling in fibromyalgia patients and are a major factor contributing to an impaired quality of life. Fibromyalgia-related headaches are either vascular, as in an autonomically mediated headache, (e.g., migraine), or are caused by muscular tension. The latter results from osteoarthritic bone spurs in the neck or from myofascial tender points or muscle spasm in the back of the neck.

Vascular headaches in fibromyalgia patients may be treated acutely with NSAIDs (see Chapter 21); *ergot alkaloids* (e.g., Ergostat, dihydroergotamine, DHE-45, Migranol); epilepsy drugs, such as *valproic acid* (Depakote); or a Tylenol, sedative, and blood-constricting combination known as Midrin. Severe headaches can be relieved with an agent that acts on the serotonin receptors, *sumatriptan* (Imitrex), *zomitriptan* (Zomig), or, if necessary, with injectable or oral narcotic analgesics such as *meperidine* (Demerol).

In addition to biofeedback and relaxation techniques, a variety of agents taken between headaches may prevent new attacks if headaches are persistent. These include *calcium channel blockers* (e.g., verapamil—Calan, Isoptin, Verelan); *tricyclic antidepressants,* such as amitriptyline (Elavil) in doses of 50–100 mg at night; and *beta blockers,* such as propranolol (Inderal). None of these preparations treat acute headaches, but when used between headaches, they prevent the development of new ones and break a headache cycle.

Muscular tension headaches are treated with NSAIDs, the muscle relaxants

Table 14. *Dr. Wallace's approach to headache in fibromyalgia patients*

1. Is the headache continuous or does it come and go?
   a. If it is continuous, obtain an MRI scan of the brain and, if the pain is in the back of the head or neck, obtain cervical spine X-rays. Is the neurologic examination abnormal? A neurologic or neurosurgical referral may be warranted if a tumor, disc, subdural bleed, abscess, aneurysm, or vascular malformation is present.
   b. If the headache is intermittent, is it a migraine (related to vascular spasm), cluster or histamine headache (related to foods or environmental factors), muscular tension headache, premenstrual, or sinus infection? If it is in the back of the neck, is it due to arthritis of the spine or to cervical muscle spasm? Is high blood pressure present?
   c. What makes the headache better or worse? Migraines are usually on one side and worsen with light exposure. Muscular tension is often associated with generalized fibromyalgia flares, and pains in back of the head improve with muscle relaxants or traction.
2. The treatment of an intermittent headache depends on its source, but a few general principles apply.
   a. Try acetaminophen or an NSAID (e.g., Aleve or Advil).
   b. If (a) is needed regularly, consider using a pain killer–muscle relaxant combination for acute, severe headaches on an occasional basis. These agents include Midrin, Esgic, Fiorinal, and Fioricet.
   c. If the therapies in (b) are needed regularly, consider ergots if migraine is present (e.g., Ergostat, Cafergot, Migranol), treat fibromyalgia systemically if muscles are very tight (e.g., Flexeril), or add physical therapy with relaxation techniques or cervical traction if neck and upper back pain is present.
   d. For severe, acute headaches that do not respond to (a), (b), or (c), the prophylactic regimens listed in (e) should be prescribed. Consider using sumatriptan (Imitrex), zomitriptan (Zomig) injections, a nasal inhaler, or nasal pills until they work. Narcotic pain killers or Demerol shots are rarely necessary.
   e. If headaches do not subside, consider therapies that prevent headaches such as a calcium-channel blocker (e.g., verapamil), TCA (amitriptyline [Elavil]), or a beta blocker (e.g., propranolol [Inderal], atenolol [Tenormin]). Refer to a neurologist to rule out less common causes of headaches or use specialized approaches.

mentioned above, and drugs known as Fiorinal or Esgic, which are combinations of aspirin or acetaminophen, a small amount of a barbiturate, and caffeine, with or without codeine. These agents are highly effective and also relieve vascular headaches. However, they are intended only for occasional use since rebound headaches may result from suddenly interrupting regular use of caffeine, aspirin, or barbiturate-containing preparations.

Pain shooting through the back of the head, or occipital headaches from tender points in the upper neck area, are treated with physical measures such as cervical traction, massage, and other relaxation techniques in addition to NSAIDs, muscle relaxants, and trigger point injections.

Table 14 demonstrates how we approach headaches in fibromyalgia.

TREATING GUT RESPONSES:
NONULCER DYSPEPSIA (HEARTBURN)
AND IRRITABLE COLON

Symptoms of heartburn, "acid indigestion," or reflux and esophageal spasm can be alleviated with several types of agents, including *antacids* (such as Maalox or Mylanta, which are weak but inexpensive), *sulcrafates* (ulcer buffers such as Carafate, which is mildly helpful), or *H2 antagonists* (cimetidine [Tagamet], famotadine [Pepcid], nizatidine [Axid], ranitidine [Zantac]), which often give only partial relief. *Proton pump inhibitors* (omeprazole [Prilosec], lansoprazole [Prevacid]) are more effective in decreasing acid production and are generally meant for short-term or intermittent use. Lastly, *prokinetic agents* (metoclopramide [Reglan], cisapride [Propulsid]) improve gut motility and decrease reflux. Make sure that your doctor tests for *Helicobacter pylori*, a common bacterial infection that can cause ulcers. There also are anecdotal suggestions that Tagamet boosts the immune system by activating B lymphocytes.

Abdominal pain, spasm, distention, bloating, and cramping are present in 30–40 percent of fibromyalgia patients. The dietary measures reviewed in Chapter 18 are helpful, but about half of these patients have severe enough symptoms to benefit, at least intermittently, from a variety of *antispasmodic* preparations that relax muscles in the intestine. These preparations include *dicyclomine* (Bentyl), the Librium derivative Librax, *hyoscyamine* (Levsin, Levbid), and even *amitriptyline* (Elavil). A combination of a mild barbiturate and a muscle relaxant (Donnatal) taken at night decreases abdominal spasms and promotes restful sleep. Magnesium-containing preparations may relieve muscle spasms as well as constipation.

MEDICATIONS THAT HELP TO MANAGE
DEPRESSION AND ANXIETY

Depression is associated with a lower pain threshold (see Chapter 4). The prevalence of depression or anxiety at any given time in fibromyalgia patients is a little under 20 percent and is over 50 percent during the course of the disorder. In our experience, 10–15 percent of fibromyalgia patients reach the point where they benefit from therapies other than those reviewed in the last chapter: TCAs, SSRIs, or benzodiazepines.

Several other families of drugs manage depression but have little, if any, influence on fibromyalgia. These include the *phenothiazines* (Thorazine, Mellaril, Prolixin, Stelazine, Risperdal, Haldol) for psychotic depression, *tricyclic-like* antidepressants (buproprion [Wellbutrin], amoxapine [Ascendin], maprotiline [Ludiomil], clomipramine [Anafranil, Mirtazapine, Remeron]) for selected patients who have specific problems not ameliorated by TCAs or SSRIs, and *monoamine oxidase inhibitors* (phenelzine [Nardil], tranylcypromine [Parnate]) used for severe depression. The latter category has specific drug or food interactions, require regular blood monitoring, and thus should be prescribed *only* in concert with treatment from a mental health professional.

Anxiety prevents fibromyalgia patients from enjoying life and functioning optimally. As noted in Chapter 21, controlled studies have shown that benzodiazepines such as *alprazolam* (Xanax) reduces this problem. However, if chronic anxiety is a problem, we prefer to prescribe nonaddictive drugs that are not sedating such as *buspirone* (Buspar). Buspar increases the availability of a selective serotonin receptor. Another useful agent is the short-acting benzodiazepine *lorazepam* (Ativan). Taken at bedtime, this drug is largely out of the system within 4 hours and helps anxious patients fall asleep.

CAN OTHER DRUGS HELP CHRONIC FATIGUE?

Of all the symptoms and signs reviewed in this chapter, patients most frequently ask for "something, anything" for fatigue. We usually use a TCA at first, since promoting restful sleep often alleviates daytime tiredness. Adding a serotonin promoter such as Prozac frequently provides an energy boost and improves symptoms of cognitive impairment.

For the remaining 15–20 percent of our patients who have significant fatigue in spite of TCA and/or SSRI therapy, we usually start with the mildest therapies and work our way up. First, we make sure that the patient is not anemic, does not have a low thyroid level, or does not have a high sedimentation rate, which would indicate systemic inflammation. As noted in Chapter 6, there are numerous nonfibromyalgia causes of fatigue that have specific treatments. Chapter 18 reviews practical, nonmedication methods to treat fatigue.

Some practitioners swear by *vitamin B_{12}* injections, which in published studies help about 20 percent of patients and are harmless. At least one study showed that patients with chronic fatigue syndrome have decreased spinal fluid levels of vitamin B_{12}, and another study demonstrated increased spinal fluid levels of a closely related chemical, homocystine. Other physicians prescribe *thyroid* even if the thyroid blood level is normal. We generally discourage this since excessive or unnecessary thyroid administration can produce a rapid heart rate and anxiety and lead to premature osteoporosis. When the patient is overweight, some doctors have tried *diet pills* (phentermine, subutramine [Meridia], over-the-counter caffeine preparations). While these agents are mild stimulants, they also can produce anxiety and palpitations. The effects of dietary suppressants frequently wear off within a few weeks to months and are not a long-term solution.

WHAT CAN BE DONE FOR COGNITIVE IMPAIRMENT WITH OR WITHOUT FATIGUE?

It was not a good year for Denise. First, her father was diagnosed with multiple myeloma, a bone marrow cancer associated with severe bone pain. At work, a new supervisor was critical of her productivity. In the spring, she had a severe case of flu with muscle and joint aches, fevers, and cough. By the time it started to ease up, Denise found that she had to sleep 10 hours a night just to make it to work, and at times she had difficulty placing names and dates. Fortunately, nobody seemed to notice. Although Dr. Denton had diagnosed her with fibromyalgia 4 years ago, Denise had not seen her in 2 years and had not taken any medication in 3 years. Trying to deal with all of her stresses seemed to make everything come back. Rather than seeing Dr. Denton, Denise consulted a "diet doctor" since she wanted to lose weight. Dr. Engel was a general practitioner who did not know what fibromyalgia was. He prescribed thyroid, vitamin B_{12} shots, and diet pills. Within a week, she was agitated and had severe palpitations. Denise's thought processes worsened, and she was unable to sleep. She returned to Dr. Denton, who told her that stress and a postviral fatigue syndrome had reactivated her fibromyalgia. Since Denise wanted to try to get by without medication, Dr. Denton referred her to a psychologist who worked with a psychiatrist. Together, they emphasized relaxation techniques and biofeedback and incorporated cognitive therapy in addition to "crisis intervention" counseling. Denise never had to take any medicine and started to feel better.

Recent studies have suggested that a hormone produced by the adrenal gland, *dehydroepiandrosteone (DHEA)*, may reduce cognitive impairment, but its mechanism of action is not clear. This agent is available from compounding pharmacies and health food stores as a food supplement and is not regulated by the FDA. We start at doses of 25–50 mg a day and sometimes go as high as 200 mg a day. Doses above 100 mg a day often produce acne and facial hair. DHEA must be used very carefully since there are reports that in men with prostate cancer or in women with early gynecologic cancer, the malignancy may become more aggressive with DHEA.

Severe cognitive dysfunction unresponsive to SSRIs may warrant a neurologic evaluation, which may include a type of brain imaging known as *SPECT scanning* (reviewed in Chapter 10). If not enough oxygen is getting to specific regions of the brain, milder amphetamine-like drugs such as *pemoline* (Cylert) are sometimes prescribed. Several published case reports have suggested that the extremely expensive calcium channel blocker *nimodopine* (Nimotop) dilates blood vessels and may improve thinking by driving more oxygen to the brain. We also have had some success with a form of counseling known as *cognitive therapy* (see Chapter 19).

Individuals in severe, vegetative states due to chronic fatigue, who cannot get out of bed for more than a few hours a day, should undergo a psychiatric evaluation and have their nutritional status evaluated. If a primary psychiatric diagnosis is ruled out, our group occasionally uses aggressive measures to help these patients function. *Fewer than 1 percent of fibromyalgia patients ever need to use any of the treatments reviewed in this paragraph.* They range from the attention-deficit disorder (ADD) amphetamine *methylphenidate* (Ritalin) and *dextroamphetamine* (Dexadrine) to the myasthenia gravis drug *pryridostigmine* (Mestinon), which promotes acetylcholine (and, indirectly, growth hormone) activity. Mestinon has been used to manage severe fatigue and cognitive impairment since the 1940s, and its efficacy was documented in early published clinical trials. However, in view of Mestinon's numerous side effects, a neurologist familiar with the drug's use should be consulted if a doctor does not have a lot of experience with it. A new mestinon-like agent, *donepezil* (Aricept), used to manage Alzheimer's syndrome, is being studied in a variety of cognitive dysfunction settings. If the patient has autoantibodies, autoimmune activity, or any evidence of inflammation, the antimalarial drug *quinacrine* is available from compounding pharmacists and may be helpful.

A POTPOURRI OF POTENTIALLY USEFUL REMEDIES

Fibromyalgia patients can have a variety of systemic complaints (see Parts III and IV) that require specific interventions. Doctors frequently treat symptomatic *mitral valve prolapse* with beta blockers such as atenolol (Tenormin) or propranolol (Inderal). *Female urethral syndrome* (irritable bladder) is managed with diazepam (Valium) or cyclobenzaprine (Flexeril) for a few nights when needed. If *interstitial cystitis* (see Chapter 14) is present, dimethylsulfoxide (DMSO) instilled directly into the bladder desensitizes bladder nerve endings and relieves pain. An effective oral agent, pentosan polysulfate sodium (Elmiron), is also available. Individuals with *allergic* tendencies may be given antihistamines, antihistamine-phenothiazine combinations (Atarax, Vistaril), H2 blockers (Tagamet, Zantac), or short courses of corticosteroids as a pill, inhaler, or nasal spray. Newer-generation antihistamines that are relatively nonsedating and do not interfere with other drugs can be prescribed (fexofenadine [Allegra], cetirizine [Zyrtec], loratadine [Claritin]). NSAIDs and occasionally a muscle relaxant, vitamin B$_6$, or a diuretic for a few days until menses begin can alleviate *PMS* complaints. Patients with *autonomic dysfunction* often respond poorly to treatment, but serious neurally mediated hypotension can be improved with fludrocortisone (Florinef) or midrodrine. We treat autonomic symptoms of burning and tingling with TCAs. Sometimes, agents that affect different parts of the ANS, such as the SNS beta blocker propranolol (Inderal), or the alpha-adrenergic promoter, clonidine, are useful. *Dizziness* is usually a form of vertigo (see Chapter 10); it responds to antihistamines or benzodiazepines.

SUMMING UP

Most fibromyalgia patients who consult a rheumatologist are started on an NSAID, TCA, SSRI, or benzodiazepine. About half of these patients have additional symptoms or signs, which may lead to the prescription of at least one of the agents reviewed in this chapter. Most of these preparations are used on an occasional or intermittent basis. Toxic or habituating drugs such as narcotic pain medications, barbiturates, or amphetamine derivatives should be prescribed rarely, and only by physicians with special training or expertise in pain management, neurology, or psychiatry. Table 15 lists the drugs reviewed in this chapter.

Table 15. *Some examples of adjunctive drugs used to manage fibromyalgia-associated conditions*

1. **Local remedies**
   Trigger and tender point injections
   Nerve blocks
   Topicals containing aspirin or NSAIDS
   Topicals containing capsaicin

2. **Muscle relaxants that are not TCAs**
   Pure muscle relaxants (e.g., orphenadrine [Norgesic], carisoprodol [Soma])
   Magnesium-malic acid combinations
   Quinine

3. **Pain killers that are not TCAs or SSRIs**
   Nonnarcotic: acetaminophen (Tylenol), NSAIDs, tramadol (Ultram)
   Nontriplicate narcotic: derivatives with codeine, propoxyphene (Darvon), hydrocodone
   (Vicodin)
   Triplicate (controlled) narcotics: morphine, oxycodone (Percodan), meperidine (Demerol), narcotic patches and pumps *

4. **Agents for nerve pain and spasm**
   Anticonvulsant derivatives (e.g., clonazepam [Klonopin], carbamezine [Tegretol], phenytoin
   [Dilantin], valproic acid [Depakote], gabapentin [Neurontin])*
   Mexiletene*
   Baclofen*
   L-Dopa*
   Other benzodiazepines (e.g., diazepam [Valium])

5. **Sleep enhancers that are not TCAs (also help vertigo)**
   Benzodiazepines (e.g., tenazepam [Restoril], florazepam [Dalmane])
   Zolpidem (Ambien)
   Antihistamines (e.g., diphenhydramine [Benadryl])
   Melatonin
   Avoid: Barbiturates, triazolam (Halcion)

6. **Headache relievers**

    For acute headaches: NSAIDs, pain killers (see no. 3 above), combinations such as Fiorinal, Esgic, Midrin, ergots, sumatriptan (Imitrex)

    To prevent headaches: calcium channel blockers (e.g., verapamil), TCAs, beta blockers

7. **Functional bowel and nonulcer dyspepsia**

    Antacids

    H2 blockers (e.g., cimetidine [Tagamet]) or sulcrafate (Carafate)

    Proton pump inhibitors (e.g., omeprazole [Prilosec])

    Prokinetic drugs (e.g., cisapride [Propulsid])

    Antispasmodic agents (e.g., hyoscyamine [Levsin])

8. **Depression and anxiety therapies that are not TCAs or SSRIs**

    Psychotic depression: phenothiazines*

    TCA- or SSRI-related agents (e.g., bupropion [Wellbutrin], maprotilene [Ludiomil])

    Monoamine oxidase inhibitors (MAOIs)*

    Antianxiety benzodiazepines (e.g., alprazolam [Xanax], lorazepam [Ativan])

    Buspirone (Buspar)

9. **Chronic fatigue and cognitive impairment therapies that are not TCA or SSRI responsive**

    Vitamin B_{12}

    Stimulants: Caffeine and amphetamine preparations*

    Related to systemic pathology: thyroid, iron, anti-inflammatory drugs

    Dehydroepiandrosterone (DHEA)

    Pyridostigmine (Mestinon)*

    Calcium-channel blockers (e.g., Nimodopine-Nimotop)*

10. **Mitral valve prolapse**

    Beta blockers

11. **Irritable bladder or interstitial cystitis that is not TCA responsive**

    Benzodiazepines

    Dimethylsulfoxide (DMSO)

12. **Premenstrual syndrome**

    NSAIDs, diuretics, analgesics

13. **Dysautonomia**

    Beta blockers

    Fludrocortisone (Florinef), midrodrine

    Clonidine (Catapres)

14. **Allergies and chemical sensitivities that are not TCA or SSRI responsive**

    Hydroxyzine (Atarax, Vistaril)

    H2 blockers (e.g., cimetidine, Tagamet)

    Nonsedating antihistamines (e.g., fexofenadine, Allegra)

    Steroid inhalers or nasal sprays

---

* Should be prescribed by an expert familiar with their use and closely monitored.

23

Behind the Hype: Unproven, Experimental, Herbal, and Innovative Remedies

Therefore the moon, the governess of floods,
Pale in her anger, washes all the air,
That rheumatic diseases do abound.
William Shakespeare (1564–1616),
A Midsummer Night's Dream
Act 2, sc. 34, l. 105

Advocates of practical though controversial lifestyle approaches have always found a sympathetic ear in the United States since the time folk practitioner Sylvester Graham's principles of health, nutrition, and fitness (in addition to inventing the Graham cracker) achieved cult status in the 1840s. Heroic, misguided therapies were administered by allopathic (mainstream) physicians throughout the 19th century. This created fertile ground for promoters of patent medicines and nostrums to those escaping organized medicine's use of leeches, cupping, phlebotomy (blood drawing) knives, and brutal laxative regimens. During the Progressive Era, medicine started to improve with the establishment of postgraduate training programs at Johns Hopkins University just before the turn of the century and the regulation of medicines as part of the Pure Food and Drug Act of 1906. The final revolution occurred when two-thirds of the medical schools in the United States closed following revelations of their inadequacies by the investigative Flexner Report funded by the Carnegie Foundation in 1910. Despite these changes, however, the appeal of alternative therapies to the American public continues unabated.

The previous two chapters have described how mainstream, organized, conventional medicine approaches fibromyalgia. Even though their therapies usually provide significant relief of symptoms and signs, traditional physicians to some extent must regard themselves as failures. In the United States, 1 person in 3 has consulted a complementary medicine practitioner. These individuals spend $15 billion a year on this approach, 10 billion of which is out-of-pocket and not reimbursed by insurance. A 1996 Canadian study found that of several hundred fibromyalgia patients, 70 percent purchased unproven over-the-counter rubs, creams, vitamins, or herbs; 40 percent sought help from alternative medicine practitioners such as chiropractors, massage therapists, homeopaths, reflexologists, or acupuncturists; and 26 percent went on special diets. Since it is logical to believe that people who are tired and hurt want to get better, it follows that some fibromyalgia patients will try anything that is not harmful to improve their medical condition. This chapter is dedicated to patients who wish to "look before they leap" into nontraditional therapies.

DOCTOR, WHAT DO YOU THINK ABOUT BRAND X?

Very few of the therapies reviewed in this chapter have been shown to be effective for treating fibromyalgia in a controlled drug trial. Some of them have been mentioned in published case reports or in a series; others have been studied in controlled trials and found to be of no benefit.

What should inquiring and potentially adventurous patients know before they try alternative or innovative treatments?

1. Ask your health care provider about any and all therapies that you would like to try. Your doctor can describe any potential risk to your health or drug interactions with your other medications.

2. Check out the credentials of the practitioner who advocates an unproven approach. Is he or she board certified in a discipline recognized by the American Board of Medical Specialties?

3. If the treatment is part of a study, make sure there is some form of informed consent listing all the risks and benefits of participating in a trial. An experimental trial should be performed at no cost to the volunteer and supervised by an Institutional Review Board.

4. If the proposed treatment is an alternative therapy that does not require approval from the FDA, such as a vitamin, food additive, or food supplement, check out the following:

   a. Have the results of this treatment been published in the medical peer-reviewed literature? Never believe testimonials, which often contain "junk science" and hearsay. Some promotional pamphlets list articles from the literature that gives them a professional or academic look, but the citations are not from any journal or book you would find in *Index Medicus*. Are the key cited papers less than 30 years old? Call the library of your nearest medical school to make sure or even obtain copies of the articles.

   b. Is the health care provider selling a remedy directly to you for profit? If so, be very skeptical of any claims. Most patients fill their prescriptions at a pharmacy, not at the doctor's office.

   c. How much is this therapy going to cost, and is it affordable?

d. How much time has to be committed to visiting the practitioner or undergoing a treatment in a setting outside the home?
e. What are the potential side effects? Does this unproven therapy require a
   lifestyle change, and is it really worth trying?
f. Do the time, effort, and cost outweigh the potential benefits? Set a limit:
   "I will try Brand X for 2 months, and if I'm not much better, forget it!"
g. What or who is the source of the promotion? Fibromyalgia patients spend
   millions of dollars a year on unproven remedies after seeing advertise-
   ments or claims in the lay press or on the Internet that enrich people they
   know nothing about. Don't be naive or gullible. If Brand X is really a
   cure, who is suppressing it or preventing the discoverer from getting a
   Nobel Prize?

ROLL CALL OF THERAPIES: FACTS, FICTION, AND FANCY

Numerous antimicrobial agents, vaccines, hormones, food supplements, and
"immune boosters" have been purported to help fibromyalgia. This section will
critically review our experience and that reported in the peer-reviewed literature
with some of these preparations.

Antibiotics and related therapies

Although *minocycline*, a derivative of tetracycline, improves mild rheumatoid
arthritis, it has no effects on fibromyalgia because the latter is a noninfectious
and non-inflammatory condition. *Poly 1, Poly CI2U (ampligen)* is an antiviral
agent potentially useful for AIDS that has been studied in chronic fatigue syndrome. This expensive intravenous preparation improved energy levels in a controversial, though controlled, study trial and is awaiting a "go-ahead" from the
FDA for further evaluations. Controlled trials showed that the antiherpes (the
herpes family includes the Epstein-Barr virus) medicine *acyclovir* (Zovirax) has
no effect on chronic fatigue syndrome. Case reports attesting that the anti-
influenza agent *amantadine* (Symmetrel) improves fatigue have not been confirmed. We are skeptical of these claims since amantadine contains an antihistamine, which causes drowsiness. *Botulinum toxin*, which in large doses is
responsible for muscle and nerve paralysis in botulism, has been injected locally
into spastic areas in small amounts, with reported improvement, and is the focus
of several ongoing studies. *Viral vaccines* have been used by a few alternative-
therapy physicians, but only a few poorly documented letters in chronic fatigue
newsletters claim success.

Yeast, or candida, is a fungus. The use of *antiyeast* preparations in the form of antifungal antibiotics (e.g., Nystatin, fluconazole [Diflucan], ketoconazole [Nizoral]) should be based on positive cultures for candida, *not* on antibodies indicating prior exposure to the fungus. Controlled studies have shown that fibromyalgia and chronic fatigue syndrome symptoms are not ameliorated by these therapies. We never prescribe antiyeast medicine unless a positive culture is present. Many antifungal preparations have potential hematologic and liver toxicity and should be regularly monitored. Yeast overgrowth, if truly present, infrequently leads to increased gas, bloating, fatigue, depression, or poor sleep habits (see Chapter 14). Using acidophilus decreases yeast by promoting the growth of good bacteria.

Hormones

Hormones are chemicals made in one organ that travel through the blood to another organ, where they have a physiologic action. As discussed in Chapters 13 and 21, systemic *steroids* often cause a flare of fibromyalgia. *Adrenal cortex* is a natural steroid made by the adrenal gland that is available without a prescription. In larger doses it acts like prednisone, which can aggravate fibromyalgia and result in dependency. Our group showed that *calcitonin*, a hormone made by the parathyroid gland, modestly reduces bone pain in fibromyalgia patients but has no effect on fatigue or muscle pain. A few patients have reported increased well-being with *bromocriptine* (Parlodel), an agent that prevents prolactin from stimulating breast milk secretion, or *oxytocin*, a hormone made by the hypothalamus that is released during labor, lactation, and orgasm. *Thymus gland* extracts are heavily promoted in Europe for their "rejuvenating" properties, none of which have been borne out in peer-reviewed controlled trials. *Growth hormone* may repair muscle microtrauma (see Chapter 5), but this expensive preparation has many other potentially toxic effects. *Pregnenolone* and natural progesterones may be useful in selected patients with cognitive impairment, moodiness, or fatigue.

Vitamins and food supplements

Vitamins and food supplements are generally safe, though totally unregulated. Testimonial claims, commission sales, and pseudoscientific tracts annually bring in hundreds of millions of dollars to resourceful entrepreneurs. For example, there is ample evidence that under the microscope *antioxidants* are capable of cleaning up oxygen-containing free radicals that damage cells. However, no antioxidant is absorbed by the gastrointestinal tract and gets into cells in sufficient quantities to have any meaningful antioxidant effect on the body. This has not stopped purveyors of food supplements and vitamins from promoting literally hundreds of harmless and useless concoctions as antioxidants that make one feel good and retard the aging process.

The roles of *chromium, mushrooms, garlic, potaba,* and *liver extracts* have never been specifically studied in fibromyalgia patients. A negative controlled trial has appeared regarding *selenium.* Patients with a rare group of muscle disorders known as *mitochondrial myopathies* may respond partially to *coenzyme Q10,* and reports have appeared suggesting that it lessens symptoms of cognitive impairment and fatigue. These preparations are very popular in Japan, where over 300 formulations are available, but controlled studies are needed.

Combinations of *free fatty acids* and *primrose oil* may decrease coronary artery disease and improve circulation, but their effects on tissue oxygenation in fibromyalgia have not been adequately studied. The late Nobel laureate Linus Pauling was a powerful advocate of megadose *oral vitamin C* supplementation in preventing infections and promoting a sense of well-being. However, we know of no evidence that expensive intravenous infusions of vitamin C are improving anything except the treating practitioner's wealth.

A by-product of vitamin B_{12} from pigs, *kutapressin,* has a cadre of alternative care physicians who swear by weekly injections, even though the only published controlled trial showed that patients who received placebo had an equal reduction in fatigue.

Amino acids, serotonin, and immune boosters

Amino acids are the building blocks of proteins. L-*threonine* may alleviate restless legs syndrome. L-*tryptophan* promotes serotonin but is potentially dangerous (see Chapters 4 and 13). A precursor of L-tryptophan, 5-hydroxytryptophan, is available from compounding pharmacies, but a controlled trial found it to be ineffective.

Ironically, an expensive antinausea drug that blocks serotonin, *ondensatron* (Zofran), was shown in a recent study to be mildly effective in fibromyalgia.

We still don't know what role, if any, the immune system plays in fibromyalgia. Even though some studies have characterized chronic fatigue syndrome as a state of too much immune activation, some practitioners advocate giving "immune-boosting" *gamma globulin* infusions to these patients. Intravenous gamma globulin infusions are very expensive ($5000 a month) preparations that modulate immune responses. Their use is restricted by hospitals and insurance companies to patients with serious immune deficiencies and certain autoimmune or neurologic disorders. A controlled trial reported that patients with chronic fatigue syndrome who received gamma globulin felt better than those receiving placebo. Other controlled trials have failed to confirm this, and the original trial's methodology has been questioned. An immune booster, *dialyzable leukocyte extract,* did not demonstrate any benefits in a clinical trial.

Guaifenesin and other odds and ends

A California internist has popularized a theory that fibromyalgia results from a defect in phosphate metabolism and its resulting effects on muscle. An extension of this hypothesis states that agents such as an expectorant found in cold medicines, guaifenesin, promote the excretion of uric acid (crystallized uric acid causes gout), which helps fibromyalgia. None of the numerous muscle studies reviewed in Chapter 5 lend any support to this line of thinking, and the theory has never been published in any peer-reviewed medical journal. In fact, Dr. Robert Bennett at the University of Oregon conducted a double-blinded, placebo-controlled, prospective trial that conclusively proved that guaifenesin is not only useless in treating fibromyalgia, it does not even promote the excretion of uric acid!

Topical salves with anesthetic or anti-inflammatory properties, such as hyaluron, gold, EMLA (eutectic mixture of lidocaine anesthetics), aurum (a combination of aspirin, camphor, and menthol), capsaicin, or quotane, may be helpful but have not been adequately studied. We reported that *hyperbaric oxygen* may improve cognitive impairment in fibromyalgia. Even though a negative controlled study was published, some doctors believe that the antidepressant *S-adenosylmethionine* may stimulate the central nervous system and help fibromyalgia. A sleeping pill not available in the United States, *zopicline*, improves sleep in the disorder but does not reduce morning stiffness, tenderness, or pain. Another sleep-promoting agent, *antidiencephalon serum*, may have modest effects. A few case reports have suggested that fibromyalgia responds to *lithium,* a drug given for manic-depressive psychosis. *Low-level laser* therapy has been delivered to painful areas with variable results. A best-seller written by a family practitioner purports that *cartilage components* such as glucosamines and chondroitin sulfate help degenerative osteoarthritis. These claims have not been adequately studied and have no theoretical relevance to fibromyalgia. One prominent chronic fatigue specialist gives his patients *nitroglycerin* under the tongue to see if temporarily improving blood flow to the brain will make any difference. Nitroglycerin frequently causes headaches. A common cough suppressant, *dextromethorphan*, in the form of Humabid LA, may inhibit the NMDA receptor pathway, which perpetuates chronic pain amplification. Intravenous *lidocaine* may temporarily relieve pain by blocking sodium channels and blocking NMDA receptors, as might the oral preparation *lamotrigine* (Lamictal).

WHAT ABOUT HERBAL REMEDIES AND HOMEOPATHY?

Seed plants that are processed and used as medicine are known as *herbs*. The use of herbs as medicine dates back thousands of years and was independently developed by hundreds of cultures throughout the world. The pharmaceutical industry, mainstream physicians, and particularly alternative-therapy physicians have studied and recommended herbal remedies for a variety of ailments. Though no herbal remedies specifically for fibromyalgia have been studied, one of my rheumatologist mentors, Dan Furst, M.D., and his wife, Elaine Furst, R.N., at the University of Washington in Seattle, have put together a useful "Herb Chart," which is reproduced in Table 16 for informational purposes. They have concluded that some herbs can be helpful, others can be harmful, and still others have no effect.

Samuel Hahnemann (1755–1843) was a physician who rebelled against the vigorous and often unsuccessful therapies promoted by his allopathic colleagues discussed at the beginning of this chapter. In response, he founded the discipline of *homeopathy*. Homeopaths administer extremely small doses of natural extracts from plants, animal products, and minerals, some of which are harmful in larger doses, in an effort to stimulate a safe chemical response or effect. Adopting a poorly understood philosophy that "like cures like" mixed in with concepts of vaccination and immunization that were years ahead of their time, users of these innocuous remedies saved many lives in the 19th century. At its peak in 1900, there were 20 homeopathic medical schools and thousands of practitioners. Homeopathy experienced a slow decline that was accelerated when its last two medical schools, New York Medical College and Hahnemann Medical College in Philadelphia, became allopathic in 1950. Over the last 10–20 years, the availability of homeopathic preparations without a prescription has sparked resurgent interest in the discipline. In 1994, $165 million was spent on these agents in the United States, and 6000 practitioners have completed training courses on how to use them. In a survey, 37 percent of family practitioners in Great Britain responded that they use some homeopathic remedies, including the Queen's physician.

Several homeopathic remedies are promoted as being helpful for arthritis and musculoskeletal pain. A few have been subjected to small, controlled trials, with contradictory results—half of them validating modest benefits. In our opinion, these agents are generally harmless, but their benefits in fibromyalgia are unproven.

ARE IMMUNIZATIONS OR ALLERGY SHOTS SAFE?

Fibromyalgia patients frequently ask whether or not they can receive routine immunizations and allergy shots out of concern for their immune system. Nothing has ever been published or reported in the peer-reviewed literature suggesting that individuals with fibromyalgia react differently to these injections than otherwise healthy people.

Table 16. *Herb Chart (for antiarthritics, skin treatments, and gastrointestinal treatments)*

Herb	Claimed Uses	Active Ingredients	Potential Side Effects
Alfalfa	Antiarthritic	Nonprotein amino acid (L-canavanine) and some saponins	In large quantities, could produce pancytopenia (decreased white blood cell count, anemia) could reactivate systematic lupus erythematosus
Arnica	Analgesic, anti-inflammatory (external application)	Sesquiterpenoid lactones (helenalin, dihydrohelenalin)	May cause contact dermatitis; cannot be taken internally; causes toxic effects on the heart and increases blood pressure
Black cohosh	Antirheumatic, sore throat, uterine difficulties	Substances that bind to estrogen receptors of rat uteri; also acetin, which causes some peripheral vasodilation	Information on toxicity is lacking; could cause uterine bleeding
Burdock	Treatment of skin conditions	Polyacetaline compounds that have bacteriostatic and fungicidal properties	Side effects may result from addition with belladonna
Butcher's broom	Improve venous circulation, anti-inflammatory	Steroidal saponins (not corticosteroids)	Unknown; self-medication for circulatory problems is dangerous
Calamus	Digestive aid, antispasmotic for dyspepsia	Unknown	Use only Type 1 (North American) calamus, which is free of carcinogenic iso a sarone (may promote cancers)
Calendula (marigold)	Facilitate healing of wounds (lacerations)	Unknown	Unknown
Capsicum	Counterirritant used to treat chronic pain (herpes zoster, facial neuralgia, or surgical trauma)	Capsaicin (proven analgesic in osteoarthritis, used externally)	Use caution in application; avoid getting into eyes or other mucous membranes; remove from hands with vinegar

[191]

Table 16. *Herb Chart* (continued)

Herb	Claimed Uses	Active Ingredients	Potential Side Effects
Catnip	Digestive, sleep aid	*Cis-trans*-nepetalactone (attractive only to cats)	Unknown; does not mimic marijuana when smoked
Chamomilles, yarrow	Aids digestion, anti-inflammatory; antispasmotic, anti-infective	Complex mixture of flavonoids, coumarins, *d*-bisabolol motricin and bisabololoxides A+B	Infrequent contact dermatitis and hypersensitivity reactions in susceptible people
Chickweed	Treatment of skin disorders, stomach and bowel problems	Vitamin C, various plant esters, acids, and alcohols	Unknown
Comfrey	General healing agent, stomach ulcer treatment	Atlantoin, tannin, and mucilage, some vitamin B$_{12}$	Hepatotoxicity (liver); can lead to liver failure, especially when the root is eaten; also causes atropine poisoning due to mislabeling
Cranberry	Treatment of bladder infections	Antiadhesion factors (fructose and unknown polymeric compounds) prevent adhesion of bacteria to lining of bladder	Increased calories if used in large doses (12–32 ounces per day) as a treatment rather than as a preventative (3 ounces per day)
Dandelion	Digestive, laxative, diuretic	Taraxacin (digestive), vitamin A	Free of toxicity except for contact dermatitis in people allergic to it
Devil's claw	Antirheumatic	Har pagoside	None
DongQuai	Antispasmotic	Coumarin derivatives	Large amounts may cause photosensitivity and lead to dermatitis, possible bleeding
Echinacea	Wound healing (external), immune stimulant (internal)	Polysaccharides, cichoric acid, and components of the alkamide fraction	None reported, but allergies are possible; be sure product is pure and not adulterated with prairie dock (can cause nausea, vomiting)

Table 16. *Herb Chart* (continued)

Herb	Claimed Uses	Active Ingredients	Potential Side Effects
Evening primrose	Treatment of atopic eczema, breast tenderness, arthritis	*Cis*-gamma-linoleic acid (GLA) (some suggestive data)	No data; borage seed oil (20% as GLA) may be a substitute and does have toxic side effects (liver toxicity, carcinogen)
Fennel	Calms stomach, promotes burping	*Trans*-anethole, fenchone, estragole, camphene, L-pinene	Do not use the volatile oil—causes skin reactions, vomiting, seizures, and respiratory problems; no side effects with use of seeds
Fenugreek	Calms stomach, demulcent	Unknown	None
Garlic	GI ailments, reduces blood pressure, prevents clots	Allin (sulphur-containing amino acid derivative), ajoene	Large doses are needed (uncooked, up to 4 grams of fresh garlic a day), which may result in GI upsets; can "thin" the blood (anticoagulant)
Gentian	Appetite stimulant	Glycosides and alkalids; increases bile secretion	May not be well tolerated by expectant mothers or people with high blood pressure (possibly increasing pressure)
Gingko biloba	Helps dementia	Antioxidant	Very well tolerated
Ginseng	Adaptogen, cure-all, anti-stress agent	Triterpenoid saponins	Be sure the product is pure; some insomnia, diarrhea, and skin eruptions have been reported; possible immune stimulant (antagonizes other medications)
Goldenseal	Digestive aid, treatment of genitourinary disorders	Alkaloids (hydrastine and berberine)	In *huge* doses, may cause uterine cramps
Honey	Sore throat, antiseptic, anti-infective, antiarthritic, sedative	Fructose, glucose, sucrose, tanin	Do not give to children under 1 year of age; may cause botulism in infants

Table 16. Herb Chart (continued)

Herb	Claimed Uses	Active Ingredients	Potential Side Effects
Lovage	Diuretic, promotes burping	Lactone derivatives (ph thalides)	Some photosensitivity with volatile oil of lovage
L-tryptophan	Sleep aid, antidepressant	Essential amino acid that increases chemical serotonin, leading to some sleepiness	Be sure product is pure; contaminants may cause a serious blood disorder and a scleroderma-like illness
Mistletoe	Stimulates smooth muscle (American); antispasmotic and calmative (European)	Phoratoxia and viscotoxin (depending on the plant species)	Berries are highly toxic, and the leaves may also cause cell death; in animals lowers blood pressure, weakens, constricts blood vessels
Nettle	Antirheumatic, antiasthmatic, diuretic, against BPH	Histamine, acetylcholine, 5-hydroxytryptamine	Skin irritation from the active ingredients
New Zealand green-lipped mussel	Antiarthritic	Amino acids, mucopolysaccharides	No toxicity or side effects except in those allergic to seafood
Passion flowers	Calmative, sedative	Unknown or disputed	None
Peppermint	Calms stomach, promotes burping, antispasmotic	Free menthol and esters of menthol	Do not give to infants and young children, who may choke from the menthol
Pokeroot	Rheumatism, cure-all	Saponin mixture (phytolaccatoxin), mitogen, pokeweed mitogen (PWM)	Vomiting, blood cell abnormalities, hypotension, decreased respiration, gastritis
Rosemary	Antirheumatic, digestive, stimulant	Camphor, borneol, cineole, diosmin (a flavonoid pigment)	Large quantities of the volatile oil taken internally cause stomach, intestinal, and kidney irritation

Table 16. *Herb Chart* (continued)

Herb	Claimed Uses	Active Ingredients	Potential Side Effects
Rue	Antispasmotic, calmative	Quinoline alkaloids, coumarin derivatives	Skin blisters and photosensitivity following contact; gastric upsets when taken internally; may be an effective antispasmotic but is too toxic to be used
St. John's wort (Hypericum)	Antidepressant, anti-inflammatory, wound healing	10% tanin, xanthones, and flavonoids that act as monoamine oxidase inhibitors (antidepressants)	Photosensitivity dermatitis in those who take the herb for extended periods; Prozac-like; increases serotonin
Sairei-to	Antiarthritic	12 herbs in combination	Diarrhea, abdominal pain, rash
Sassafras	Antispasmotic, antirheumatic	Safrole	Active ingredient is carcinogenic in rats and mice
Senna	Cathartic	Dianthrone glycosides (sennosides A+B)	Diarrhea, gastric, and intestinal irritation with large and/or habitual doses
Tea tree oil	Antiseptic (external application only)	Terpene hydrocarbons, oxygenated terpenes (terpinen-4-ol)	No side effects except skin irritation in sensitive individuals
Valerian (garden heliotrope)	Tranquilizer, calmative	Unknown	None noted
Yucca	Antiarthritic	Saporins	None noted

Source: Compiled by Elaine E. Furst, R.N., and Daniel E. Furst, M.D. Modified from V. E. Taylor: The Honest Herbalist, 3 ed., Binghamton, NY: Haworth Press, 1993, pp. 336–351.

[195]

SUMMING UP

Few of the preparations mentioned in this chapter have proven efficacy in managing fibromyalgia. However, some of these agents are being studied in controlled trials and may prove useful in the future. Patients of ours have had favorable experiences with St. John's wort and gingko biloba. Here's some friendly advice. Don't be talked into taking any preparation mentioned in this chapter without consulting a fibromyalgia specialist who is certified by a recognized specialty board. Let the buyer beware!

24
Work and Disability

Fibromyalgia patients are not disabled; they are differently abled.

Adapted from James McGuire, M.D.
(1949–1997), rheumatologist

Most of us have to work for a living. There are bills to pay and families to provide for. Since fibromyalgia patients do not usually look ill and on superficial examination appear strong, complaints of difficulty performing the job can be hard to believe. This chapter will review definitions as they apply to disability, impairments reported in fibromyalgia patients, and constructive approaches that allow individuals with the syndrome to work most effectively.

LET'S COME TO TERMS: WHAT IS DISABILITY?

The World Health Organization defines *disability* as a limitation of function that compromises the ability to perform an activity within a range considered normal. Efforts to manage work disabilities considers issues such as age, sex, level of education, psychological profile, past attainments, motivation, retraining prospects, and social support systems. Additionally, work disability issues take into account work-related self-esteem, motivation, stress, fatigue, personal value systems, and availability of financial compensation.

An *impairment* is an anatomic, physiologic, or psychological loss that leads to disability. Impairments include pain from work activities (e.g., heavy lifting), emotional stress (e.g., working in a complaint department), or muscle dysfunction (e.g., cerebral palsy). A *handicap* is a job limitation or something that cannot be done (e.g., deafness).

Patients with a disability can be *permanently, totally disabled* and thus potentially eligible for Social Security Disability and Medicare health benefits. Other classifications include being *permanently, partially disabled*, whereby vocational rehabilitation, occupational therapy, and psychological or ergonomic evaluations can address impairments or handicaps to optimize employment retraining possibilities. *Temporary, partial disability* allows one to work with restrictions (e.g., no lifting more than 10 pounds) while treatment is in progress. *Temporary, total disability* involves a leave of absence from employment while undergoing treatment so that one can return to work.

Subjective factors of disability include symptoms such as pain or fatigue, while objective factors of disability are physical signs such as a heart murmur or a swollen joint. One can be disabled from a *work category* and granted disability even if employment is ongoing in a different work category. Work categories are rated as sedentary, light work, light medium work, medium work, heavy work, or very heavy work, each defined by how much exertion is used over a time interval. Additional consideration is given to repetitive motions such as bending, squatting, walking up stairs, and squeezing, as well as environmental temperature or the operating of heavy equipment.

DO MOST FIBROMYALGIA PATIENTS WORK?

In the United States, up to 90 percent of fibromyalgia patients who wish to work are able to do so. Sixty percent of fibromyalgia patients are working full time. (The other 30 percent are housewives, househusbands, and retirees.) In a 7-university center study of 1500 individuals with fibromyalgia, 25 percent had received disability payments at some time, and 15 percent received Social Security Disability (and Medicare) benefits. As noted before, studies from university medical centers include patients who have more severe problems and do not reflect the patient population seen in community-based rheumatology practices. Despite this, two-thirds of academic-based study patients related that they were able to work nearly all the time.

However, these statistics are deceiving and do not relate the problems fibromyalgia patients have had with employment. For example, in another survey, 30 percent of these patients had to change their jobs due to the disorder, and 30 percent modified their jobs in some way to accommodate their symptoms. All told, in the United States at any time, 6–15 percent of employed fibromyalgia patients are on some form of disability. In nations with more generous disability systems such as Sweden, up to 25 percent of these patients are considered disabled.

WHY ARE SOME FIBROMYALGIA PATIENTS DISABLED?

The most common reason fibromyalgia patients say they cannot work is severe pain. This creates many problems because pain is a subjective sensation that is hard for others to understand. After all, employers point out, other employees with pain are able to work. Additional factors that limit employment in fibromyalgia patients include poor cognitive functioning (inability to think clearly), fatigue, stress, and cold, damp work environments. Fibromyalgia patients complain of having decreased stamina or endurance and frequently have poor body mechanics. This limits their ability to undertake repetitive lifting, bending, or squatting, assume unnatural positions, or use excessive force. Using standardized test measurements in a study of light to medium jobs that required repetitive movements, fibromyalgia patients performed only 58.6 percent of the work done by healthy co-workers. This may be due to a decrease of up to one-third in muscle strength per unit for repetitive activities in patients with the syndrome. Interestingly, there is a discrepancy between perceived work ability and what is viewed on videos of work performance. Most fibromyalgia patients perform better than they think.

Another important factor relates to psychological makeup. Patients unable to deal with pain, low self-esteem, a strong feeling of helplessness, and low educational levels have a worse outlook.

Do fibromyalgia patients malinger, or make up their symptoms for purposes of secondary (such as monetary) gain? Although offers of financial compensation are always attractive, several studies have shown that over 90 percent of the time, fibromyalgia does not stop working after litigation is settled. In Israel, where work disability is not recognized, trauma is associated with the same prevalence of postinjury fibromyalgia as in the United States. On the other hand, an epidemic of fibromyalgia-related "repetitive strain disorder" in the late 1980s in Australia was eliminated by minor changes in regulations.

WHAT RIGHTS DOES A FIBROMYALGIA PATIENT HAVE?

The Americans with Disabilities Act protects individuals from job discrimination by requiring companies with more than 15 employees to make adjustments ("reasonable accommodations") for people with disabilities and chronic illnesses. These modifications include having an occupational therapist or ergonomic expert evaluate the work site. If fibromyalgia is brought on or aggravated by poor body mechanics or emotional stress caused at work, individuals are eligible for medical treatment, disability, and job retraining through the workers compensation system. Accommodations include part-time or half-day employment or a leave of absence. Most medium-sized and large companies have private disability policies. Although these approaches are all too often abused, their intent is to keep disabled people employed. If the disability is total and permanent, many individuals are eligible for Social Security benefits. Fibromyalgia, however, is not considered a disabling condition by the U.S. government. Therefore, the small number of patients with fibromyalgia who are totally, permanently disabled are usually granted Social Security benefits on the basis of related conditions such as chronic fatigue, pain, arthritis, or depression—all accepted disabilities under government rules.

HOW CAN TOTAL DISABILITY BE PREVENTED?

Vicki was a crack systems analyst whose computer skills got her jobs, but she never seemed able to keep them. Over a 5-year period, Vicki had accepted but had been terminated or resigned from 5 separate positions. She had a long-standing diagnosis of fibromyalgia, which was adequately controlled with a combination of cyclobenzaprine (Flexeril) in the evening and sertraline (Zoloft) in the morning. Vicki encountered numerous problems in trying to hold her jobs: an inability to work overtime when certain projects demanded it, feeling faint when co-workers smoked around her, dealing with terrible chairs and glare at her computer workstations, snickers from co-workers when she took midday breaks, disputes with her boss when she tried to get time off to see her doctor, and being forced to lift 20-pound file boxes. Vicki became defensive, and a bad attitude got her fired from her last job before she completed the probation period. Through her fibromyalgia support group, Vicki was put in contact with an occupational therapist who consulted part-time on workstation ergonomics for a Fortune 500 company. With the help of the occupational therapist and a vocational rehabilitation counselor, Vicki put together a résumé showing how productive her work could be and the potential benefits for the company that exploited her creative talents. At her next job interview, Vicki appeared very positive but made it clear that the potential employer would have to recognize her partial disability. By making a few minor modifications to her work schedule, alterations that involved no cost to the company, she could become an outstanding worker. Vicki has now held her job for 3 years, loves every minute of it, and recently was promoted.

Despite all that has been related in this chapter, almost 90 percent of fibromyalgia patients in the United States who wish to work can be employed in some capacity.

In this section, we'll review strategies that enable patients to minimize pain and function as productively as possible.

Find an agreeable environment

Try to find a workplace that is quiet and smoke free, has clean air or is well ventilated, is adequately lit, and has a comfortable noise level.

Be up front and positive with your employer

If fibromyalgia alters work performance or may require workstation or workplace modifications, let the employer know about the syndrome but do it in a positive way. Relate all the things you *can* do and how your productivity can be enhanced with minimal accommodations.

Pace yourself

Learn to manage time and prioritize job responsibilities and obligations. Make sure that a work day has several rest periods and a reasonable lunch break, which helps minimize fatigue. Focus your energy on what is important. Have a positive attitude and learn to laugh.

Strategize and use coping skills

Co-workers should be made aware of whatever adaptations are necessary for optimal productivity so that they will not view these as perks or become jealous. Learn to cope with the office environment—you cannot fire the boss. Don't get stressed out about what cannot be changed or about policies you do not control.

Examine the workstation

It is important to limit or avoid excessive lifting, reaching, twisting, standing, bending, overhead use of arms, and squatting. Consider using supportive braces or bands when engaging in these activities. Alternatively, follow employee manuals or physician or allied health professional (e.g., physical or occupational

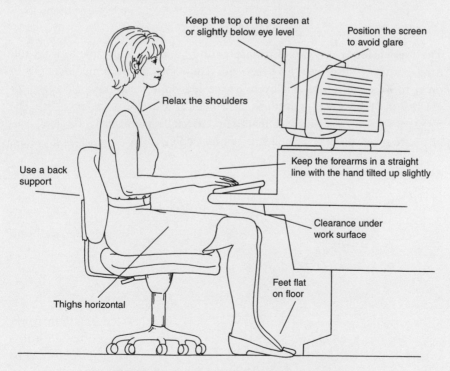

Fig. 23 *An ergonomically correct workstation.*

therapist) instructions if these motions are necessary for the job, since it's necessary to minimize harm from work trauma.

Make sure your chair has a firm back and does not compress the circulation. Its height and back should be comfortable and at the right level for your computer keyboard. If the job requires heavy telephone use, consider using a speakerphone or headset to minimize neck and upper back strain.

Follow the recommendations in the computer manual regarding height, monitor angle, type of chair to be used, and screen glare. Keep arms parallel to hips, the hands above the keyboard and even or below the elbows, wrists straight, and fingers curved; special keyboards or soft pads may be helpful. When typing, arms should hang comfortably from the shoulders. The shoulder should be relaxed and not scrunched. An example is shown in Figure 23.

Help yourself

Maintain correct posture to ease muscle strain, learn to relax, and keep physically conditioned. Take short work breaks to deep-breathe, relax, and stretch. Patients who have difficulty coping or who notice worsening pain shouldn't keep things to themselves. Call a doctor, mental health advisor, or physical therapist.

SUMMING UP

The overwhelming majority of patients with fibromyalgia are able to work full time, but up to 40 percent may have to change jobs or make modifications in order to be productively employed. These individuals may take advantage of existing disability laws, protections, and medical resources to achieve this. The 5–10 percent of fibromyalgia patients who are totally, permanently disabled usually have severe problems with pain, fatigue, coping skills, or depression.

Part VIII
WHERE ARE WE HEADED?

We're the first to agree that the fibromyalgia therapies reviewed in the previous two sections are far from perfect. However, they are a long way from "You'll just have to learn to live with it"—advice most doctors offered just a few years ago. The good news is that there are a lot of developments on the horizon. This part discusses the outcomes of fibromyalgia and presents a baseline from which physicians and researchers are working toward improvements. Many new approaches for treating fibromyalgia are the focus of well-designed studies, some of which will make substantial differences in the quality of life for fibromyalgia patients in the near future.

25

What's the Prognosis?

*Diseases desperate grown. By desperate appliances are
relieved. Or not at all.*

William Shakespeare (1564–1616),
Hamlet, Act 4, sc. 3, l. 9

When patients are diagnosed with fibromyalgia, one of their first questions to us
relates to its outcome. "Is there hope, doc?" and "Will the pain ever go away?"
are two of the more common queries we hear. Unfortunately, few surveys have
addressed this issue, and those that have arrived at contradictory conclusions.
This chapter will try to put these studies in their proper perspective. Yes, there is
hope!

WHAT HAPPENS TO MYOFASCIAL PAIN SYNDROME?

When discomfort is limited to a specific region of the body and is not widespread, the outlook for long-term relief of pain is usually quite good. With local
physical measures, injections, emotional support, and anti-inflammatory and
analgesic medication, as well as instruction in proper body mechanics, over 75
percent of regional myofascial pain syndrome patients have substantial pain
relief within 2–3 years. Unfortunately, there is little middle ground. For example,
in an 18-year analysis of 53 patients with low back pain followed by musculoskeletal specialists, 25 percent ultimately developed fibromyalgia. Therefore,
we believe that myofascial pain should not be shrugged off or given short shrift.
A problem that is addressed early and effectively saves patients, health plans, and
society money. Also ameliorated are the heartaches of patients and those close to
them. Improved productivity promotes a feeling of relief, as well as a better quality of life. When a practitioner prescribes Advil and says that this is all that can
be done for TMJ dysfunction syndrome, it is penny wise but pound foolish.

WHAT HAPPENS TO FIBROMYALGIA?

The outcome of fibromyalgia depends on who sees the patient and calls the
shots. For example, in one report that tracked family practitioners, internists, or
other primary care physicians familiar with fibromyalgia's diagnosis and man-

agement, 24 percent of patients were in remission at 2 years and 47 percent no longer met the ACR criteria for the syndrome. This implies that early intervention by a knowledgeable community physician is the first line of therapy. Children with fibromyalgia also have a favorable outcome. In the largest study to date, symptoms resolved in 73 percent within 2 years of diagnosis.

The outlook in tertiary care settings is not as rosy. Once the symptoms and signs of the syndrome are serious enough to warrant referral to an academically oriented rheumatologist who is involved in fibromyalgia research, improvement is common but recovery rare. A summary of academic-based studies suggests that at 3 years, 90 percent of patients still have symptoms. They were rated as moderate to severe in 60 percent of the cases, and only 2 percent were cured. Among these patients, measures of pain, disability, function, fatigue, sleep, and psychological health change disappointingly little over the years. Those who fulfill the criteria for chronic fatigue syndrome tend to get better if they can trace their disease onset to an infection. Among this grouping, two-thirds are improved at 2 years. In our community rheumatology practice, we frequently find that most patients feel better after they are educated about the syndrome and treated. Many generally do well, but if the weather changes, a new emotionally stressful situation occurs, or physical trauma is sustained, relapse may occur. However, since these patients are connected to a rapid-response medical environment, long-term damage or disability can be prevented.

CAN A BAD OUTCOME BE PREDICTED?

Several investigators have tried to find unifying characteristics of patients who failed to respond to treatment. These individuals tended to have severe mood or behavioral disturbances, received less than 12 years of formal education, or were older than 40 when their symptoms began. In our experience, patients who are psychotic (those who carry the diagnosis of schizophrenia, bipolar disease, paranoia, or delusional disorder) or are not successfully treated for substance abuse do not improve.

WHAT CAN PATIENTS DO TO IMPROVE THEIR OUTLOOK?

In the United States, too many health plans provide too much "tough love." As a result, fibromyalgia patients must be their own advocates. Patients with the syndrome should seek a practitioner who knows what fibromyalgia is, believes that it exists, and wants to help people with the disorder. If a health plan restricts access to this type of physician, patients should reiterate that nearly all health plans are required to provide the best possible care for specific problems. If this care is not available within a certain environment, the insurer must make accommodations to do the best for the subscriber's health and well-being. We're not talking about breaking the bank! A 6-center survey of 538 chronic fibromyalgia patients treated in an academic setting (and, by definition, having more severe disease) had an average medical bill of $2274 a year over a 7-year period. Fibromyalgia patients rarely benefit from surgery or hospitalization for their condition. With the assistance of their fibromyalgia caregiver, patients may need to supply their carrier with evidence supporting the need for physical therapy, occupational therapy, vocational rehabilitation, cognitive therapy, or psychological counseling in order for their symptoms to improve. Patients can help themselves further by joining the Arthritis Foundation, subscribing to fibromyalgia support group newsletters, and keeping abreast of advances in the field. Informed, motivated patients who help themselves ultimately feel better and have an improved quality of life.

THE BOTTOM LINE

If fibromyalgia is identified early and managed appropriately, patients usually improve. Patients who know what fibromyalgia is and are motivated to improve their condition fare better than passive individuals who get lost in the bureaucracy of our medical establishment. In our experience, it's harder for patients to improve (though not impossible) if therapy is delayed for more than 5 years. Individuals who are psychotic, or who are addicted to drugs or alcohol, will not improve until their psychiatric and emotional problems are addressed first.

26
The Future Holds A Lot of Hope

The future has waited long enough; if we do not grasp it,
other hands, grasping hard and bloody, will.

Adlai Stevenson (1900–1965)
to Murray Kempton, 1963

When we became interested in fibromyalgia 20 years ago, we quickly learned how it felt to be lonely. The Fibrositis Study Club (now the Fibromyalgia Study Club) of the American Rheumatism Association (now the American College of Rheumatology) had an average attendance of 10 at its annual meetings. In 1997, more than 500 rheumatologists attended the same meeting. In the early 1980s, an average of 14 articles a year appeared in the fibromyalgia medical literature, and less than $100,000 was being spent annually on fibromyalgia research. The recognition of fibromyalgia by organized medicine as a distinct syndrome has had a salutary effect on research. As of this writing, 300 articles are now published yearly and $2 million is spent annually on research. All this attention and interest bodes well for more scientific breakthroughs in the field. What can fibromyalgia patients hope for over the next 20 years?

AN IMPROVED CLASSIFICATION

In all probability, the name *fibromyalgia* will be replaced by a more all-encompassing term, one that includes related syndromes that have similar causes and physiologic processes. A better (and catchier) term than *dysregulation spectrum syndrome*, which combines symptoms and signs reported in tension headache, pain amplification, irritable bowel syndrome, irritable bladder, and chronic fatigue syndrome, among others, will be devised and agreed on. When organized medicine marshals the resources of experts in gastroenterology, infectious disease, rheumatology, and other subspecialties to work together, our knowledge of pain amplification, neurotransmitter-mediated, behaviorially influenced fatigue syndromes will be increased, and research strategies will be better coordinated and focused. Fibromyalgia advocacy groups will unite to increase funding for research and education that will make a difference.

We predict that 2–5 percent of the U.S. population will have a dysregulatory spectrum syndrome. Over the next 20 years, the precise racial and ethnic backgrounds of these individuals will be identified, as well as the genes that influence the process. Additionally, environmental and occupational factors that cause or aggravate the process will be clarified. Through coordinated strategies involving all forms of media, the public will become aware of what fibromyalgia is and what factors are associated with it. Increased awareness through an updated medical education curriculum will allow health care practitioners to intervene earlier to treat patients who develop fibromyalgia symptoms or signs after an injury or infection. This, in turn, will improve the prognosis and outcome. Better support systems will be available for individuals who require all forms of counseling or job retraining through the Arthritis Foundation and fibromyalgia support organizations.

BASIC RESEARCH ADVANCES

In the next decade, we predict that the body's pain pathways will be better demarcated and understood. Feedback loops and the source of what stimulates or suppresses certain "wires" or nerves will be elucidated. The roles of substance P, serotonin, the ANS, epinephrine, endorphin, dopamine, and other important chemicals that affect mood, pain perception, and transmission of information from one region to another will be better defined. For example, if we can block messages sent by excitatory amino acids (which amplify chronic pain but play no role in acute pain), a new class of drugs that specifically treats fibromyalgia pain can be formulated.

The nervous system does not work in a vacuum but involves interactions with hormones, the immune system, muscles, sleep, and stress factors. The biology of cytokines and other groups of chemicals that interrelate these components will be better understood. Along these lines, investigators will be able to answer several important questions in the next 20 years. Why are some behavior patterns associated with pain amplification but not others? Does muscle spasm result from a local reflex or does it come from signals within the spinal column? What does sleep have to do with growth hormone? Is there anything wrong with the immune system of fibromyalgia patients? Why do reflexes within the ANS increase numbness, tingling, flushing, headaches, cramping, and burning rather than help people with fibromyalgia? How do viruses or other microbes cause chronic fatigue syndrome? What really goes on inside a local tender point?

PHYSICAL AND PSYCHOLOGICAL INTERVENTIONS

Coordinated efforts will improve physician education and lead to diagnostic testing or imaging that will provide practitioners with readily available tools to confirm the diagnosis of fibromyalgia. Skeptical health care professionals will no longer refer to fibromyalgia as a "wastebasket" or the "emperor's new clothes" disease. Once a diagnosis is confirmed, our nonmedication approaches will be fine-tuned. For example, as more allied health professionals are trained in cognitive therapy, fibromyalgia patients will be able to think better and function with greater mental clarity. Information about physical therapy measures that are harmful in fibromyalgia but useful in other forms of musculoskeletal disease will be better disseminated once more therapists take an Arthritis Foundation certification course detailing specific approaches that do and do not benefit fibromyalgia patients. Exercise and conditioning programs currently being developed will be tested, widely available, and reimbursed by third-party carriers. Ergonomics will play a greater role in the prevention of fibromyalgia as companies find that it is in their interest to have healthy, productive, motivated, pain-free employees working at comfortable workstations. The next editions of the *Diagnosis and Statistical Manual for Mental Disorders* (*DSM*), used for psychiatric diagnosis, will confront the dysregulatory spectrum syndrome directly and create a new category for pain amplification. In turn, emphasis will be put on how to improve self-esteem, decrease pain perception, and deal with the reactive depression and anxiety related to fibromyalgia. This information will be incorporated into the training of mental health professionals (e.g., psychologists, social workers, counselors, clergy, psychiatrists).

FIBROMYALGIA THERAPIES: THE NEXT GENERATION

Current medications used to manage fibromyalgia will be improved. Newer, less toxic ibuprofen and aspirin-like drugs will be on the market in the next few years with the development of cyclooxygenase-2 antagonists. Safer and more specific TCAs (e.g., Elavil-like) and SSRI (e.g., Prozac-like) agents are on the horizon. Benzodiazepines (e.g., Klonopin-like) with less potential for inducing depression or addiction will be introduced. Vaccines against fibromyalgia-inducing infections may become available.

New classes of medicines will block substance P; increase serotonin or adenosine A; release more endorphins; modulate calcium-magnesium in muscle channels or sodium channel blockers in cells; and block excitatory amino acids, nerve growth factor, and dynorphins. Agents that stabilize the ANS will be developed as our knowledge of cell signaling and cell surface receptors evolves. Biochemistry and neurochemistry advances will allow for the development and introduction of medications that act as kinin receptor antagonists, nitric oxide synthetase receptor antagonists, and tachykinin receptor antagonists and analogues of capsaicin. All of these preparations potentially are capable of decreasing pain and diminishing pain perception. Over the next 20–30 years, gene manipulation and control over apoptosis (programmed cell death) will challenge ethicists and scientists as we become capable of fundamentally manipulating our genes, cells, and progeny—thus, perhaps, greatly reducing the properties and production of pain.

Fibromyalgia patients should not give up hope. We've come so far in the last decade. Now, new exciting challenges are just beginning!

Glossary

acetaminophen (Tylenol) a mild pain reliever occasionally useful in fibromyalgia.

acetylcholine a neurotransmitter of the autonomic nervous system (see below) that induces dilation of blood vessels and slows down the gastrointestinal and urinary tracts.

acupuncture traditional Chinese medicine therapy that reduces pain by inserting very fine needles just under the skin at points along "life force" pathways called meridians.

acute of short duration and coming on suddenly.

adrenal glands small organs, located above the kidney, that produce many hormones, including corticosteroids and epinephrine.

adrenalin see epinephrine.

aerobic exercise designed to increase oxygen consumption.

affective spectrum disorder a term used to consider irritable bowel, tension headache, irritable bladder, premenstrual tension, and fibromyalgia as being primarily of behavioral and secondarily of physiologic causation.

afferent nerves nerves going from the periphery (e.g., skin, muscle) toward the spine.

alexithymia long-standing personality disorder with generalized and localized complaints in individuals who cannot express underlying psychological conflicts.

allodynia what happens when something that should not hurt causes pain. Fibromyalgia is chronic, widespread allodynia.

alpha/delta sleep wave abnormality delta waves make up most of slow wave, or nondream, sleep. Alpha waves interrupting delta waves can produce movement or awakening, leading to unrefreshing sleep.

American College of Rheumatology (ACR) a professional association of 5000 American rheumatologists and 2000 allied health professionals (the Association of Rheumatology Health Professionals).

analgesia decreased perception of pain.

anemia a condition resulting from a low red blood cell count.

ankylosing spondylitis an inflammatory arthritis of the spine, sacroiliac, and sometimes peripheral joints. Most patients have a positive HLA-B27 blood test.

anti-inflammatory   an agent that decreases inflammation.

antinuclear antibody (ANA)   proteins in the blood that react with the nuclei of cells. Found in 96 percent of patients with lupus and in up to 10 percent of those with fibromyalgia.

artery   a blood vessel that transports blood from the heart to the tissues.

arthralgia   pain in a joint.

arthritis   inflammation of a joint.

Arthritis Foundation   a nonprofit national organization that provides patient support and funds research on musculoskeletal disorders.

aspirin   an anti-inflammatory drug with pain-killing properties.

autonomic nervous system (ANS)   part of the peripheral nervous system and divided into sympathetic and parasympathetic components. Regulates stress responses, sweat, urine, and bowel reflexes and determines if a blood vessel constricts or dilates, thereby affecting pulse and blood pressure.

B cell   a white blood cell that makes antibodies.

benzodiazepine   a potentially addictive group of drugs, including Valium and Klonopin, that relaxes muscles, among other actions, by blocking GABA (see below).

biofeedback   a training technique enabling an individual to gain some voluntary control over autonomic body functions.

biopsy   removal of tissue for examination under the microscope.

body dysmorphic disorder   a condition of individuals engrossed with themselves who express excessive concern or fear over having a defect in appearance.

bradykinins   chemicals that mediate inflammation and dilate blood vessels.

bruxism   persistently grinding one's teeth.

bursa   a sac of synovial fluid between tendons, muscles, and bones that promotes easier movement.

candida hypersensitivity syndrome   a controversial condition based on theories that a toxin released by yeast is responsible for irritable bowel, fatigue, and a feeling of illness. Candida is a type of yeast, or fungus.

capillaries   small blood vessels that connect arteries to veins.

carpal tunnel syndrome   compression of the median nerve as it traverses the palmar side of the wrist, producing shooting nerve pains in the first to fourth fingers.

cartilage   tissue material that covers bone.

causalgia   sustained burning pain, allodynia, and overreaction to stimuli associated with autonomic nervous system dysfunction. Reflex sympathetic dystrophy is chronic, widespread causalgia.

Centers for Disease Control (CDC)   an agency of the federal government based in Atlanta that monitors, defines, and sets standards for managing epidemics, infections, new diseases, and certain types of blood tests.

central nervous system   nerve tissue in the brain and spinal cord.

chiropractic   a therapy involving manipulation of spine and joints to influence the body's nervous system and natural defense mechanisms.

chronic   persisting for a long period of time.

chronic fatigue immune dysfunction syndrome (CFIDS)   a controversial term for chronic fatigue syndrome implying a prominent role for immune abnormalities.

chronic fatigue syndrome (CFS)   unexplained fatigue lasting for more than 6 months associated with musculoskeletal and systemic symptoms. Most of these patients fulfill the criteria for fibromyalgia.

cognitive behavioral therapy   the use of biofeedback-related techniques to improve speech and memory.

cognitive dysfunction   difficulty focusing, remembering names or dates, performing numerical calculations, or articulating clearly.

collagen   structural protein found in bone, cartilage, and skin.

complete blood count (CBC)   a blood test that measures the numbers of red blood cells, white blood cells, and platelets in the body.

computed tomography (CT)   a method of imaging a region of the body using a specialized type of X-ray.

conversion reaction   a form of hysteria whereby an emotion is transformed into a physical manifestation (e.g., a person with normal vision claiming that "I can't see").

corticosteroid   any anti-inflammatory hormone made by the adrenal gland's cortex, or center.

corticotropin-releasing hormone (CRH)   a chemical made in the hypothalamus of the brain that ultimately leads to the release of steroids by the adrenal gland.

cortisone   a synthetic corticosteroid.

costochondritis   irritation of the tethering tissues connecting the sternum (breastbone) to the ribs, producing chest pains; also called Tietze's syndrome.

cytokines   messenger chemicals of the immune system.

dehydroepiandrosterone (DHEA)   a hormone made by the adrenal cortex and also by the testes with male hormone properties.

delta sleep   a type of electrical wave found on a tracing of brain waves during nondream sleep.

depression   helplessness and hopelessness leading to feelings of worthlessness, loss of appetite, alterations in sleep patterns, loss of self-esteem, inability to concentrate, complaints of fatigue, and loss of energy.

disability   a limitation of function that compromises the ability to perform an activity within a range considered normal.

dorsal horn   nerves inside the back of the spinal cord. Runs from the brain to the waist area.

dorsal root ganglion   nerve cell bodies in the peripheral nervous system that receive nociceptive inputs and transmit them to the spinal cord.

dynorphin   an opiate that suppresses acute pain but perpetuates chronic pain.

dysautonomia   abnormal function of the autonomic nervous system.

dysfunction   partial, inadequate, or abnormal function of an organ tissue or system.

dysmenorrhea   painful periods.

edema   swelling of tissues, usually due to inflammation or fluid retention.

efferent nerves   nerves that go from the spinal cord to its periphery.

electroencephalogram (EEG)   a mapping of electrical activity within the brain.

electromyogram (EMG)   a map of electrical activity within muscles. Usually combined with a *nerve conduction velocity* study, which assesses nerve damage or injury.

endorphin   chemical substance in the brain that acts as an opiate. Relieves pain by raising the body's pain threshold.

enkephalin   similar to endorphin (see above).

enzyme   a protein that accelerates chemical reactions.

eosinophilia myalgic syndrome (EMS)   a scleroderma-like thickening of fascia (see below) associated with high levels of circulating eosinophils caused by a contaminant of L-tryptophan. Many patients with EMS develop fibromyalgia.

eosinophilic fascitis   a form of EMS (see above) probably induced by excessive shunting of L-tryptophan from the serotonin (see below) pathway to an alternative pathway.

epidemiology   study of relationships between various factors that determine who gets a disorder and how many people have it.

epinephrine   or adrenalin, a "nerve hormone" produced in the adrenal gland that acts as a neurotransmitter and stimulates the sympathetic nervous system.

Epstein-Barr virus (EBV)   a herpesvirus producing a mononucleosis-like illness that can lead to chronic fatigue syndrome.

ergonomics   a discipline that studies the relationship between human factors, the design and operation of machines, behavior, and the physical environment.

erythrocyte sedimentation rate (ESR)   see sedimentation rate.

estrogen   female hormone produced by the ovaries.

exacerbation   reappearance of symptoms; a flare.

excitatory amino acids such as glutamate and aspartate function as neuro-transmitting chemicals in chronic pain. When they are blocked, fibromyalgia pain is relieved.

fascia a layer of tissue between skin and muscle.

fatigue feeling weary or sleepy; may lead to reduced efficiency of work, accomplishment, or concentration.

female urethral syndrome irritable bladder; persistent urge to void without evidence of infection, obstruction, stricture, or inflammation.

fever a temperature above 99.6°F.

fibromyalgia chronic, widespread, amplified pain associated with fatigue, sleep disorder, tender points, and systemic symptoms.

fibrositis an outdated term for fibromyalgia (see above); discarded since it implies inflammation, which is usually not present.

flare reappearance of symptoms; another word for exacerbation.

gamma-aminobutyric acid (GABA) an inhibitory neurotransmitter.

gate theory blocking or regulating transmission of pain impulses in the dorsal horn of the spinal column.

gene consisting of DNA, it is the basic unit of inherited information in our cells.

Gulf War syndrome a fibromyalgia-like disorder among Gulf War (1991) veterans probably caused by taking a combination of medicines meant to protect them from chemical warfare.

handicap a job limitation; something that cannot be done.

homeopathy a discipline based on the idea that symptoms can be eliminated by taking infinitesimal amounts of substances that, in large amounts, would produce the same symptoms.

hormones chemical messengers made by the body, including thyroid, steroids, insulin, estrogen, progesterone, and testosterone.

hyperalgesia exaggerated response to a painful stimulus.

hypermobility laxity of ligaments allowing one to assume positions or undertake movements difficult for a normal person to do.

hyperpathia delayed or persistent pain from noxious stimuli.

hypochondriasis excessive preoccupation with the fear of having a serious disease based on misinterpretation of one or more bodily symptoms or signs.

hypoglycemia low blood sugar level.

hypothalamic-pituitary-adrenal (HPA) axis the system by which a releasing hormone secreted by the hypothalamus induces the pituitary gland to secrete stimulating hormone, which, in turn, induces the adrenal glands to release steroid-related hormones.

hypothalamus a region of the brain that produces chemicals which result in the release of hormones.

hypoxia   insufficient oxygen reaching a tissue, organ, or region of the body.

hysteria   see conversion reaction.

immunity   a body's defense against foreign substances.

impairment   an anatomic, physiologic, or psychological loss that leads to disability.

incidence   the rate at which a population develops a disorder.

inflammation   swelling, heat, and redness resulting from the infiltration of white blood cells into tissues.

interferon   sugar-protein substances with antiviral activity that can produce cognitive impairment with aching.

interleukin   sugar-protein substances that are intercellular mediators of inflammation and the immune response.

interstitial cystitis   a chronic inflammatory condition of the bladder.

irritable bladder   see female urethral syndrome.

irritable bowel syndrome   symptoms of abdominal distention, bloating, mucus-containing stools, and irregular bowel habits without an obvious cause.

joint   the articulation between two bones.

leaky gut syndrome   a controversial entity based on the belief that an overload of poisons overwhelms the liver's ability to detoxify, making the intestinal lining more permeable.

ligament   a tether attaching bone to bone, giving them stability.

limbic system   a collection of brain structures that influences endocrine and autonomic systems and affects motivational and mood states.

livedo reticularis   a lace-like pattern of small veins and capillaries visible on the skin.

lupus   (also systemic lupus erythematosus [SLE]) an autoimmune multisystemic disease caused by abnormal immune regulation resulting in tissue damage.

Lyme disease   caused when a deer-borne tick infects people with a bacterium; it is frequently associated with fibromyalgia and fatigue syndromes.

lymphadenopathy   swollen, palpable lymph nodes.

lymphocyte   type of white blood cell that fights infection and mediates the immune response.

magnetic resonance imaging (MRI)   a picture of a body region derived from using magnets; involves no radiation.

melatonin   a substance made by the pineal gland of the brain that promotes sleep.

migraine   a vascular headache.

mitral valve prolapse   a floppy heart valve that can produce palpitations.

multiple chemical sensitivity syndrome   a controversial condition suggesting that chemicals in the environment produce symptoms and signs at levels not thought to be harmful.

muscle a primary tissue consisting of specialized contractile cells that give strength to the body.

myalgia pain in the muscles.

myelinated fibers a fat-protein sheath surrounding nerve fibers.

myoclonus twitching of a muscle or a group of muscles.

myofascial pain discomfort in the muscles and fascia.

myofascial pain syndrome fibromyalgia-like pain limited to one region of the body; also known as regional myofascial pain.

narcotics an opiate-derived substance that suppresses pain.

National Institutes of Health (NIH) a federal government organization that funds medical research.

neurally mediated hypotension low blood pressure due to autonomic dysfunction.

neurokinins substances made by nerves having physiologic effects.

neuropathic pathology produced by compression, damage or destruction of a nerve.

neuropeptides consist of short chemical sequences common to amino acids (a building block of protein) that have effects on one's perception of pain and can act as neurotransmitters.

neuroplasticity central brain sensitization that, if prolonged, produces phantom limb pain.

neurotransmitters chemical substances that transmit messages through nerves.

nerve conduction velocity (NCV) measures the rate of nerve transmission and is usually part of an electromyogram (see above).

NMDA (N-methyl-D-aspartate) receptor a neurotransmitter sensor or receptor different from opiates that interacts with excitatory amino acids (see above).

nociceptor a nerve that receives and transmits painful stimuli. Nociception is the process that transmits stimuli from the periphery (skin, muscles, tissues) to the central nervous system.

nonrestorative sleep waking up feeling unrefreshed.

nonsteroidal anti-inflammatory drugs (NSAIDs) agents such as aspirin, ibuprofen, or naproxen that fight inflammation by blocking the actions of prostaglandin.

norepinephrine a "nerve hormone" produced in the adrenal gland that acts as a neurotransmitter and stimulates the autonomic nervous system.

obsessive-compulsive disorder (OCD) persistent ideas or impulses; can include performing repetitive acts or perfectionistic tendencies.

occupational therapy   uses ergonomics in designing tasks to fit the capabilities of the human body.

opiates   narcotics.

organic   due to a physiologic dysfunction as opposed to a psychological disorder.

orthopedist   a doctor who operates on the body's musculoskeletal structures.

osteoarthritis   a degenerative disease of the joints related to destruction of or defects in cartilage.

osteopath   a physician who is trained in performing specialized physical manipulative modalities.

osteoporosis   loss of calcium from normal bone creating thin bones at risk of fracture.

overuse syndrome   pain in muscles, ligaments, tendons, or joints from excessive activity in an area of the body.

pain   an unpleasant sensation or emotional experience.

palindromic rheumatism   intermittent swelling or inflammation of joints.

palmar erythema   redness of the hands due to an autonomic reaction.

parasympathetic nervous system   a division of the autonomic nervous system that blocks acetylcholine.

paresthesia   a sensation of numbness, tingling, burning, or prickling anywhere in the body.

pathogenic   causing disease or abnormal reactions.

peripheral nervous system   nerves to and from the spinal cord that transmit sensation and motor reflexes.

physiatrist   a practitioner of physical medicine (see below).

physical medicine   a medical specialty concerned with the principles of musculoskeletal, cardiovascular, and neurologic rehabilitation.

physical therapist   allied health professional that assists patients with physical conditioning.

pituitary   a gland in the brain that assists in the production of hormones.

placebo   a pill or treatment that has no physiologic actions or effect; a "sugar pill."

plasma   the fluid portion of blood.

pleura   a sac lining the lung.

pleuritis   inflammation or irritation of the lining of the lung.

polymyalgia rheumatica   an autoimmune disease of the joints and muscles seen in older patients with high sedimentation rates who have aching in their shoulders, upper arms, hips, and upper legs.

polymyositis   an autoimmune, inflammatory disorder of muscles.

positron emission tomography (PET)   an imaging technique that measures the flow of a substance to tissues. Requires a cyclotron to perform.

prednisone; prednisolone   synthetic steroids.

premenstrual syndrome (PMS) the release of chemicals prior to menstruation, causing fluid retention, alterations in mood and behavior, and sometimes painful periods.

prevalence the number of people who have a condition or disorder per unit of population.

primary fibromyalgia syndrome fibromyalgia of unknown cause.

prolactin a hormone that stimulates the secretion of breast milk.

prostaglandins physiologically active substances present in many tissues.

protein a collection of amino acids. Antibodies are proteins.

psoriatic arthritis inflammatory disease of the joints in patients with psoriasis.

psychogenic rheumatism complaints of joint pain for purposes of secondary gain.

psychosomatic when parts of the brain or mind influence functions of the body.

rapid eye movement (REM) sleep the part of sleep in which we may dream.

Raynaud's disease Isolated Raynaud's phenomenon (see below); not part of any other disease.

Raynaud's phenomenon discoloration of the hands or feet (which turn blue, white, or red), especially with stress or cold temperatures; a feature of many autoimmune diseases.

reactive hyperemia increased blood flow to an area following prior interruption or compromise of circulation.

receptor area on a cell that receives chemical stimulation to activate a particular function.

referred pain perceived as coming from an area different from its actual origin.

reflex sympathetic dystrophy (RSD) a type of fibromyalgia associated with sustained burning pain and swelling.

reflexology a form of alternative medicine based on the theory that specific areas of the ears, hands, and feet correspond to organs, glands, and nerves.

regional myofascial syndrome fibromyalgia pain limited to one region of the body; also known as *myofascial pain syndrome*.

Reiter's syndrome inflammation of the joints, conjunctivitis, mouth ulcers, and a psoriasis-like rash in patients who have a positive HLA-B27 blood test.

remission a quiet period free from symptoms but not necessarily representing a cure.

repetitive strain syndrome when repetitive motions in a work environment produce strain or stress on an area of the body, as in carpal tunnel syndrome from excessive typing.

restless legs syndrome   legs that suddenly shoot out, lift, jerk, or go into spasm. If this occurs during sleep, it is called sleep myoclonus.

rheumatic diseases   any of 150 disorders affecting the immune or musculoskeletal systems.

rheumatoid arthritis   chronic disease of the joints marked by inflammatory changes in the joint-lining membranes, which may give positive results on tests of rheumatoid factor or antinuclear antibody.

rheumatologist   an internal medicine specialist who has completed at least a 2-year fellowship studying rheumatic diseases (see above).

scleroderma   an autoimmune disease featuring rheumatoid-type inflammation, tight skin, and vascular problems (e.g., Raynaud's disease).

seasonal affective disorder   when light deprivation during winter months produces depression and fatigue.

sedimentation rate   test that measures the rate of fall of red blood cells in a column of blood; high rates indicate inflammation or infection.

selective serotonin reuptake inhibitor (SSRI)   a class of drugs such as Prozac that treat depression and pain by boosting serotonin levels.

serotonin   a chemical that aids sleep, reduces pain, and influences mood and appetite. Derived from tryptophan and stored in blood platelets.

serum   clear liquid portion of the blood after removal of clotting factors.

Sicca syndrome   dry eyes. Can be due to decreased sympathetic nervous system activity, medication or Sjogren's syndrome (see below).

sick building syndrome   allergy and fibromyalgia-like symptoms complained of by more than one person with extreme sensitivity to environmental components in the same home or workplace.

sign   an abnormal finding on a physical examination.

silicone   a synthetic organopolymer used in liquid form in breast implants and in solid form in joint replacements and intravenous tubing.

siliconosis   controversial syndrome implying that leakage of silicone from breast implants is responsible for systemic symptoms.

single photon emission computed tomography (SPECT)   a less sophisticated PET scan (see above) that does not require a cyclotron. In fibromyalgia it can diagnose cognitive dysfunction by documenting insufficient oxygen reaching the brain.

Sjogren's syndrome   dry eyes, dry mouth, and arthritis observed in many autoimmune disorders or by itself (primary Sjogren's).

sleep myoclonus   restless legs syndrome (see above) that occurs during sleep.

slow wave sleep   a phase of sleep not associated with dreaming but with alpha waves on an electroencephalogram (see above).

soft tissue rheumatism   musculoskeletal complaints relating to tendons, muscles, bursa, ligaments, and fascial tissues. Includes fibromyalgia.

somatization conversion of anxiety and other psychological states into physical symptoms.

somatomedin C a form of growth hormone.

somatotropin growth hormone.

spasm increased muscular tension or involuntary muscular contraction.

spinoreticular tract a trail of nerves that conducts impulses to the brain that regulate the autonomic nervous system from the periphery.

spinothalamic tract a trail of nerves that conveys impulses to the brain associated with touch, pain, and temperature.

steroids shortened term for corticosteroids, which are anti-inflammatory hormones produced by the adrenal gland's cortex or synthetically.

substance P a neurotransmitter chemical that increases pain perception.

sympathetic nervous system (SNS) a branch of the autonomic nervous system that regulates the release of norepinephrine (see above).

symptoms a subjective complaint relating to a bodily function or sensation.

syndrome a constellation of associated symptoms, signs, and laboratory findings.

synovitis inflammation of the tissues lining a joint.

synovium tissue that lines the joint.

systemic pertaining to or affecting the body as a whole.

systemic lupus erythematosus see lupus.

taut band a tight, rubber-band-like knot in the muscles.

T cell a lymphocyte responsible for immunologic memory.

temporomandibular joint (TMJ) dysfunction syndrome pain in the jaw joint associated with localized myofascial discomfort.

tender point an area of tenderness in the muscles, tendons, bony prominences, or fat pads.

tendon structure that attaches muscle to bone.

thalamus an oval mass of gray matter in the brain that receives signals from nerve tracts in the spinal cord.

thyroid a gland in the neck that makes a hormone that helps to regulate the body's metabolism.

Tietze's syndrome another term for costochondritis (see above).

tinnitus ringing in the ears.

titer amount of a substance.

toxic oil syndrome a form of eosinophilia myalgic syndrome (see above) caused by adulterated cooking oil.

tricyclic a family of antidepressant drugs such as Elavil that relieve depression, promote restful sleep, relax muscles, and raise the pain threshold.

trigger point an area of muscle that, when touched, triggers a reaction of discomfort.

tryptophan   an amino acid that can be broken down to serotonin.

urinalysis   analyzing a urine sample under the microscope.

vaginismus   tightness of the vaginal muscles, which prevents or limits penetration during sexual intercourse.

vasculitis   inflammation of the blood vessels.

vertigo   malfunction of the vestibular (balance center) of the ear, producing a sensation that everything around you is in motion.

visceral hyperalgesia   pain amplification mediated by the parasympathetic nervous system thought to cause irritable bowel and ulcer-like symptoms.

vocational rehabilitation   training someone for an occupation, which takes into account the person's educational background and physical skills, as well as his or her handicaps or impairments.

vulvodynia   pain in the female genital area when infection, cancer, stricture, or inflammation has been ruled out.

yeast   a type of fungus.

Appendix 1
Fibromyalgia Resource Materials

Many resources are available to fibromyalgia patients. The listings below are not intended to be inclusive or exhaustive, but represent sources within the United States that the authors have found useful to their patients. Several of the fibromyalgia books mentioned below have more comprehensive information about source materials.

WHAT OTHER BOOKS CAN I READ ABOUT FIBROMYALGIA?

Arthritis Foundation. *Your Personal Guide to Living Well with Fibromyalgia* (Longstreet Press, Atlanta, GA, 1997, 221 pages). Translates their highly popular self-help course into readable prose.

Backstrom, G., and B. Rubin. *When Muscle Pain Won't Go Away,* revised edition (Taylor Publishing, Dallas, TX, 1995, 185 pages). Presents an osteopathic perspective.

Fransen, J., and I. J. Russell. *The Fibromyalgia Help Book: Practical Guide to Living Better with Fibromyalgia* (Smith House Press, St. Paul, MN, 1996, 239 pages). Offers worksheets and practical suggestions that help patients help themselves.

Goldenberg, D. L. *Chronic Illness and Uncertainty. A Personal and Professional Guide to Poorly Understood Syndromes* (Dorset Press, Newton Lower Falls, MA, 1997, 226 pages). A sensitive personal account by a gifted fibromyalgia investigator.

Goldstein, J. A. *Betrayal by the Brain: The Neurologic Basis of Chronic Fatigue Syndrome, Fibromyalgia, and Related Neural Disorders* (Haworth Medical Press, Binghamton, NY, 1996, 272 pages). Details the author's limbic system hypothesis, which might explain what produces fibromyalgia.

McIlwain, H. H., and D. F. Bruce. *Fibromyalgia Handbook* (Henry Holt and Co., New York, 1996, 194 pages). Broadly outlines approaches that help rheumatic disease patients.

Pellegrino, Dr. Mark. Dr. Pellegrino is a physical medicine specialist who has published several tracts that emphasize correct body mechanics, including *The Fibromyalgia Survivor* (119 pages), *Understanding Post-traumatic Fibromyalgia* (130 pages), and *Fibromyalgia: Managing the Pain* (84 pages), that are periodically updated and added to. A current listing is available from Anadem Publishing, Columbus, OH. Tel: 614-262-2539.

Pillemer, S. R., ed. *The Fibromyalgia Syndrome. Current Research and Future Directions in Epidemiology, Pathogenesis and Treatment* (Haworth Medical Press,

Binghamton, NY, 1994). A summary of the proceedings of the first National Institute of Health conference on fibromyalgia.

Starlanyl, D., and M. E. Copeland. *Fibromyalgia and Chronic Myofascial Pain Syndrome* (New Harbinger Publications, Oakland, CA, 1996, 401 pages). Long, eclectically organized, passionate tome by a family physician that combines outstanding insights with uncritical acceptance of controversial remedies and approaches.

Williamson, M. E. *Fibromyalgia: A Comprehensive Approach* (Walker Publishing Co., New York, 1995, 216 pages). Useful perspectives on the syndrome written by a fibromyalgia patient.

WHAT ARE THE BEST PAMPHLETS OR BROCHURES THAT SUCCINCTLY EXPLAIN WHAT FIBROMYALGIA IS?

Edinger, B. *Coping with Fibromyalgia*, 1991, 38 pages, and *Treating Fibromyalgia*, 1996, 50 pages, available from most fibromyalgia organizations.

Fibromyalgia Network (see listing below). *The Fibromyalgia Syndrome*. A similar pamphlet with the same name is available from the Arthritis Foundation (see listing below).

Melvin, J. L., *Fibromyalgia Syndrome. Getting Healthy*, American Occupational Therapy Association, 1996, 54 pages.

Russell, I. J. *Fibromyalgia Syndrome: A Primer*, 1996, available from most fibromyalgia organizations.

I HAVE A MEDICAL BACKGROUND. HOW CAN I KEEP UP WITH DEVELOPMENTS IN THE FIELD?

The *Journal of Musculoskeletal Pain* and *Pain* publish more peer-reviewed fibromyalgia articles than any other journal. Some of the best work in the field appears in the *Journal of Rheumatology*, *Scandinavian Journal of Rheumatology,* and *Arthritis and Rheumatism*. Join the Fibromyalgia Network and subscribe to their newsletter.

WHAT ORGANIZATIONS PROVIDE INFORMATION TO FIBROMYALGIA PATIENTS AND UNDERWRITE RESEARCH?

American College of Rheumatology (ACR), 1800 Century Place, Suite 250, Atlanta, GA 30345-4300. Tel: 404-633-377. The professional organization to which nearly all rheumatologists belong. The ACR̃s Research and Education Foundation has supported fibromyalgia research.

American Fibromyalgia Foundation, 6252 Silverwood Dr., Huntington Beach, CA 92647. Tel: 714-840-8038. Provides patient and educational support, as well as physician referrals, especially in Southern California.

Arthritis Foundation. 1300 West Peachtree St., Atlanta, GA 30309-2904. Tel: 404-872-7100 or 800-283-7800. Funds fibromyalgia research, publishes pamphlets on fibromyalgia, organizes fibromyalgia support groups and community lectures, and teaches the Fibromyalgia Self-Help Course.

Fibromyalgia Alliance of America, P.O. Box 21990, Columbus, OH. Tel: 614-457-4222. Provides patient education and publishes *Fibromyalgia Times*. Another organization with the same name is located at P.O. Box 16600, Washington, DC. Tel: 202-310-1818.

Fibromyalgia Association of Greater Washington, 12210 Fairfax Towne Center, Fairfax, VA 22033. Tel: 703-790-2324. Promotes patient education and publishes the newsletter, *Fibromyalgia Frontiers*.

Fibromyalgia Network, P.O. Box 31750, Tucson, AZ 85751-1750. Tel: 520-290-5508 and 800-853-2929. Publishes several useful brochures and the best newsletter in the country updating research and advocacy efforts. Has a physician referral list. Also supports research through the American Fibromyalgia Syndrome Association, Tel: 520-290-5550.

National Fibromyalgia Research Association, P.O. Box 500, Salem, OR 93708. Tel: 503-588-1411. Underwrites research and educational support for fibromyalgia.

National Institute of Arthritis, Musculoskeletal and Skin Diseases (NIAMS), P.O. Box AMS, 9000 Rockville Pike, Bethesda, MD. Coordinates governmental fibromyalgia funding efforts. Their information clearinghouse number is 301-495-4484.

Many states and large communities have their own fibromyalgia support organizations.

WHAT ARE THE BEST FIBROMYALGIA VIDEOS?

Many videos are available, but two that we feel are particularly useful and available from most of the eight organizations listed above are:

Fibromyalgia and You, produced by Dr. I. Jon Russell
Fibromyalgia Stretch Video, produced by Sharon Clark, Ph.D.

ARE THERE OTHER ORGANIZATIONS THAT DEAL WITH FIBROMYALGIA-ASSOCIATED DISORDERS?

Yes. There are hundreds. A few important ones are listed here.

American Academy of Physical Medicine and Rehabilitation, One IBM Plaza #2500, Chicago, IL 60611. Tel: 312-464-9700. The professional organization that physiatrists belong to.

American Holistic Health Association, P.O. Box 17400, Anaheim, CA 92817-7400. Tel: 714-779-6152. Coordinates efforts of chiropractors, osteopaths, acupuncturists, naturopaths, reflexologists, homeopaths, and massage therapists, among others.

American Occupational Therapy Association, 1383 Piccard Dr., Rockville, MD 20850, Tel: 301-948-9626.

American Osteopathic Association, 142 E Ontario St., Chicago, IL 60611. Tel: 312-280-5800.

The CFIDS Association of America (Chronic Fatigue and Immune Dysfunction Syndrome), P.O. Box 220398, Charlotte, NC. Tel: 800-442-3437.

Lupus Foundation of America, 1300 Piccard Dr., Suite 200, Rockville, MD 20850. Tel: 301-670-9292.

National Headache Foundation, 5252 N. Western Ave., Chicago, IL 60625. Tel: 800-843-2256.

Scleroderma Foundation, Peabody Office Building, 1 Newbury St, Peabody, MA 01960. Tel: 800-722-HOPE.

Sjogren's Syndrome Foundation, 335 N. Broadway, Jericho, NY 11753. Tel: 516-933-6365.

WHAT ABOUT WEB SITES, DISABILITY AND ADVOCACY GROUPS RELATING TO FIBROMYALGIA?

Fibromyalgia Web sites are always being added and change frequently. If you wish an updated current listing of Web sites, or need to find out about your disability rights or how to increase awareness of the syndrome, contact any of the eight organizations listed earlier in this section.

Appendix 2

Fibromyalgia: A Complementary Medicine Doctor's Perspective

Soram Singh Khalsa, M.D.

Soram Singh Khalsa, M.D., is a board-certified internist who chairs the Executive Steering Committee of the Complementary Medicine Program at Cedars-Sinai Medical Center in Los Angeles. A graduate of Yale University, Dr. Khalsa is a founding member of the American Holistic Medical Association, the American Academy of Medical Acupuncture, and serves on the board of directors of the Institute of Functional Medicine.

I appreciate this opportunity to present the complementary medicine clinician's perspective on the treatment of fibromyalgia. Complementary medicine is being used by an increasing percentage of Americans. In an article published in the *New England Journal of Medicine* in 1993, Dr. David Eisenberg stated that approximately one in three people in America had obtained treatment using complementary medicine over the course of a single year. Since that time, more and more Americans are using the modalities of complementary medicine, and there is increased coverage of this form of medicine in magazines and newspapers throughout the country.

Complementary medicine includes many of the modalities mentioned in this book, including chiropractic, osteopathy, nutritional medicine, herbology and homeopathy, and many others. In my practice of medicine, I often use the term *functional medicine* to describe what I do. The Institute of Functional Medicine has created a formal definition: "Functional medicine is a field of health care focused on the assessment and early intervention into the improvement of physiological, cognitive/emotional, and physical functioning." The objective is to assess individual uniqueness and implement programs using diet, lifestyle practices, and activities tailored to the person's need to promote health, resilience, vitality, and performance. There is no illness more relevant to these goals than fibromyalgia.

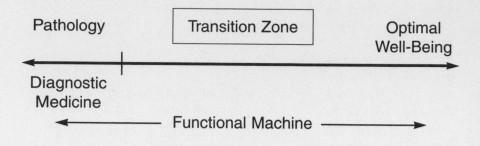

Fig. 24 *The spectrum of health*

The primary focus of complementary medicine is the concept of the spectrum of health (see Fig. 24). At one end of the spectrum of health are diseases with pathology in which tissue change and/or organ damage are detectable with blood tests, X-rays, and pathology reports. At the opposite end of the spectrum is optimal well-being. Between these extremes is a transition zone. In the transition zone, organs show no signs of pathology, yet a patient can have many symptoms. In this zone, organs begin to lose their functional reserve and do not function ideally. The goal of functional medicine is to understand where patients fall on this spectrum. Almost always, unless fibromyalgia is a component of a pathologic disease such as lupus, patients with fibromyalgia fall in the central transition zone of this spectrum of health. Many medical problems in this central zone include an interaction of dysfunctions of the immune, endocrine, neurologic, hepatic, and gastrointestinal systems. As this book clearly points out, with its interaction between the endocrine, immune, and autonomic nervous system, fibromyalgia is one such illness.

In functional medicine, we use the concept put forth by Dr. Leo Galland that there are *antecedents*—including genetic susceptibility, aging, and nutritional insufficiency—combined with specific *triggers* in our environment that include not only a physical trauma but also food antigens and toxins, xenobiotics, endotoxins, and psychological or physiologic stress. This combination of antecedents and triggers leads to the mediators, discussed in this book, that produce the inflammatory response. These include the inflammatory cytokines, including cyclooxygenase and lipoxygenase, as well as the nitric acid cytokines. These inflammatory mediators directly affect the intermediate organs of the nervous, immune, gastrointestinal, and hepatic systems. They also produce oxidative stress, which further influences these systems. This creates dysfunction in these systems, which results in the symptoms that we see in the muscular, nervous, and endocrine systems in fibromyalgia.

Dr. Wallace is correct in saying that as yet there are no formal studies proving the relationship of dysfunctional gastrointestinal function and hepatic detoxification to fibromyalgia. We do know, however, that increased permeability of the lining of the gastrointestinal tract (sometimes called *leaky gut*) is a factor in some autoimmune illnesses, including ankylosing spondylitis and rheumatoid arthritis. Many factors, including abnormal intestinal flora, can contribute to this increased permeability. Every day in my practice and in those of hundreds of my colleagues who practice as I do, we find abnormalities in these functions in patients with fibromyalgia. By correcting them, we frequently achieve major improvements in the patient's symptoms. Formal studies to document and prove this need to be done. In my role as chairman of the Steering Committee of the Cedars-Sinai Complementary Medicine Program, I plan to facilitate such studies.

Herbs, acupuncture, and homeopathy must be understood as agents used to reduce the dysfunction of the intermediate organs. Using them in combination can result in a potentiation of their effects—a result superior to that achieved by any one of the modalities alone. Although acupuncture is commonly thought of for its use in pain control, its major use is in supporting organ function. Vitamins and other nutritional cofactors including a variety of phytonutrients are used to help modify the inflammatory process, reduce intermediate inflammatory cytokines, and reduce the activity of the arachidonic acid cascade, thereby leading to reduced inflammation and the relief of pain. Specific nutritional cofactors, including the omega-3 family of fatty acids (as found in flaxseed oil and fish oil) need to be studied for their role in suppressing T-helper-1 cell production, thereby ameliorating the cause of inflammation. One such clinical trial has been published, showing the use of eicosapentaenoic acid (EPA) and docosahexaenoic acid (DHA) in inflammatory disorders such as inflammatory bowel disease, rheumatoid arthritis, and psoriasis. Such studies need to be done to see if these nutritional cofactors can be equally effective in modulating inflammation in fibromyalgia. In my clinical experience, they can indeed be useful.

In my practice with the very ill fibromyalgia patient, I endeavor to develop an overview of all the antecedents, triggers, and mediators involved, and to evaluate the functional integrity of the gastrointestinal, hepatic, and antioxidant systems of the body. By targeting therapy to the dysfunctional organs and modifying the specific triggers in the patient's environment, very gratifying clinical results are usually obtained.

By using this integrated approach to improving the functioning of the body's organ systems, there is one very interesting surprise. Most of us are familiar with the concept of *psychosomatic* influence, whereby the mind can produce effects in the body. In my many years of treating fibromyalgia, I have observed the *somatopsychic* effects of complementary medical treatment. Specifically in the case of fibromyalgia, I often find that by strengthening organ function through the modalities mentioned above, a patient's mental and emotional state can dramatically improve. Commonly in my practice, patients are able to reduce or sometimes eliminate their use of psychotropic medications as their physiology improves. This idea of somatopsychic effects needs to be studied much further. It has been observed frequently by many of my colleagues as well.

One of the problems in studying disorders in the transition zone of the spectrum of health is that there is no specific organ pathology. Rather, problems in this area are usually a complex of multiple organ system dysfunctions without disease. It is for this reason that the traditional medical study, which looks at only one variable and its effect on a target symptom, tends not to show the effectiveness of a single nutritional, herbal, or other complementary interaction. In the functional medicine approach to illness, several therapies are usually administered at once. For this reason, I believe that only outcome studies will be able to document the clinical effectiveness of most complementary forms of therapy. Medical outcome studies are more focused on function than on disease. This is very important in illnesses such as fibromyalgia. Specifically, medical outcome studies look at physical functioning, physical role, bodily pain, general health and vitality, and social functioning, as well as emotional role and mental health. These are the most important considerations in illnesses such as fibromyalgia, rather than simply looking at a result of one laboratory study, which the double-blind, crossover, placebo-controlled model of most current medical studies facilitates.

I believe that in the future we will see a new medical world where, increasingly, collaboration between traditional medical doctors and complementary medical doctors, as well as the variety of other complementary practitioners, including chiropractors, acupuncturists, herbologists, homeopaths, and osteopaths, will facilitate patient outcomes. In this way, we can begin to prove and document, in ways acceptable to all practitioners and patients, the effectiveness of these complementary modalities and the benefits of their integration with traditional medicine for the patient's health. After all, that is why all health care practitioners have embarked on their profession. This cooperation among practitioners and integration of care will lead to the improvement of patient outcomes and, in my opinion, will be especially effective in transitional zone illnesses, of which fibromyalgia is a most important example.

Index